Visual atlas of oral and dental pathologies in cats

For this English edition:

Visual atlas of oral and dental pathologies in cats
Copyright © 2017 Grupo Asís Biomedia, S.L.
Plaza Antonio Beltrán Martínez nº 1, planta 8 - letra I
(Centro empresarial El Trovador)
50002 Zaragoza - Spain

First printing: September 2017

This book has been published originally in Spanish under the title:
Atlas visual de patologías dentales y orales en pequeños animales y exóticos
© 2008 Grupo Asís Biomedia, S.L.
ISBN Spanish edition: 978-84-935971-6-0

Translation:
Anna Frandsen

Reviewed by:
Javier Collados Soto

Illustrator:
Jacob Gragera Artal

ISBN: 978-84-17225-09-4
D.L.: Z 1325-2017

Design, layout and printing:
Servet editorial - Grupo Asís Biomedia, S.L.
www.grupoasis.com
info@grupoasis.com

Servet is the publishing house of Grupo Asís

Warning:

Veterinary science is constantly evolving, as are pharmacology and the other sciences. Inevitably, it is therefore the responsibility of the veterinary surgeon to determine and verify the dosage, the method of administration, the duration of treatment and any possible contraindications to the treatments given to each individual patient, based on his or her professional experience. Neither the publisher nor the author can be held liable for any damage or harm caused to people, animals or properties resulting from the correct or incorrect application of the information contained in this book.

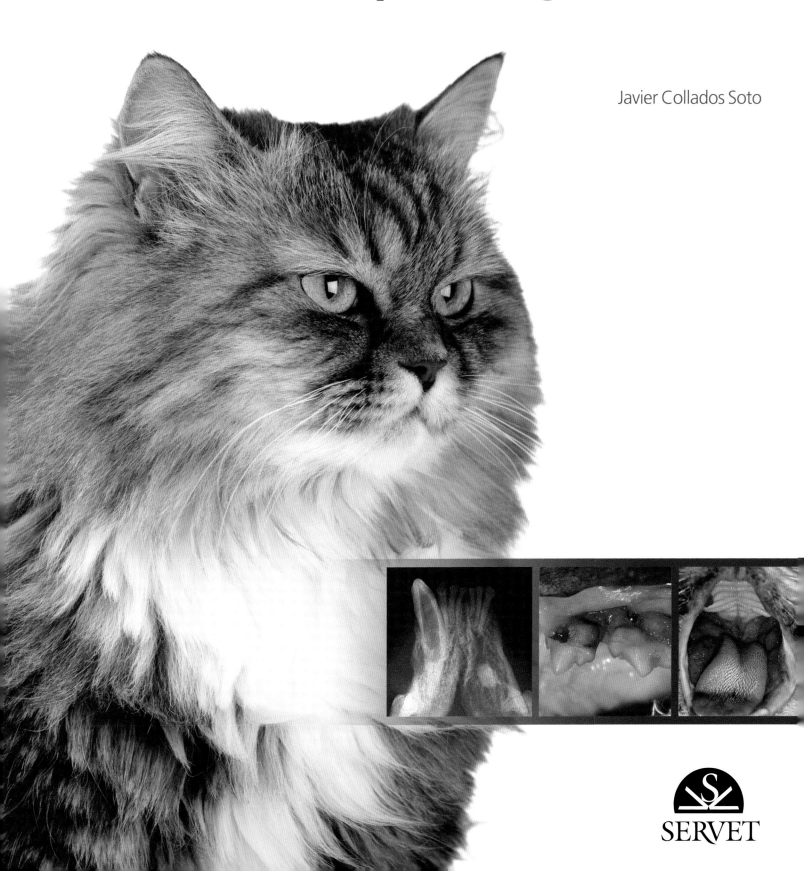

Visual atlas of oral and dental pathologies in cats

Javier Collados Soto

SERVET

This book is dedicated to my daughter Marta.

You are my best memories from the past, my dearest moments of the present, and my best wishes for the future.

Acknowledgements

To my parents, Carlos and Pilar, whose support made it possible for me to develop my skills in the veterinary world, by encouraging from the very first moment their child's dream to become a vet. To my brother David, who has always shared his knowledge of Human Dentistry with me, thus making me grow professionally in my specialty.

To my colleagues Nacho, Belén, Yolanda, Javier, Ramón, Sergio, Bea and Buzz, for showing me every day what it means to be a good vet, in its deepest and broadest concept. Especially to Luis, of whom I still keep a moving memory, and who was a living example of the profession's dignity.

To Mª Esther, an example of extreme dedication to aniwal welfare and a faithful representative of the great concept of the responsability of being a pet owner, with each and every implication this has.

To all the exceptional collaborators of the book, Antonio, Beatriz, Carlos, Carmen, Manuel, María Paz, María, Valentina and very particularly to Vittorio, for the great effort and dedication shown and expressed, all of them have made this work very important to me.

To Elena F., for her extraordinary histopathological diagnoses.

To each and every one of my vet colleagues who have believed in my particular vision of Veterinary dentistry in the last thirteen years, whose names I do not list for fear of forgetting any of them and not acknowledging him or her. This Atlas is because of and for them.

To Tao, Ciro, Brenda, Lis, Athia, Arnold, and so many other spontaneous collaborators who are part of who I really am.

To Servet, especially to Yolanda and Carlos, for their patience and excellent professionalism. I hope they are as proud of this work as I am.

To Frank, I will always consider him my mentor, and I wish to express here my most sincere gratitude to him.

Javier Collados

The author

Javier Collados Soto graduated in Veterinary Medicine from the Complutense University of Madrid (UCM) in 1994. Specialising exclusively in Veterinary Dentistry and Oral Surgery, he works in numerous veterinary practices and hospitals in Spain, concentrating his services in Madrid. He is responsible for the Dentistry and Oral Surgery service at the Sierra de Madrid Veterinary Hospital. He was a lecturer and subject coordinator in Animal Dentistry at the Faculty of Veterinary Medicine of the Alfonso X el Sabio University of Madrid.

Always showing his interest for his specialisation, he has had several stays at the Dentistry and Oral Surgery Service of the University of California (UCDavis) Veterinary Medical Teaching Hospital, USA.

He has been member of the European Veterinary Dental Society (EVDS) since 1999 and he is also one of the founder members of the Spanish Society of Veterinary Experimental Dentistry and Maxillofacial Surgery (SEOVE, *Sociedad Española de Odontología-Cirugía Maxilofacial Veterinaria y Experimental*).

He has published many articles in this specialty and has participated as a speaker in congresses and national and international courses in the field of Veterinary Dentistry.

Collaborators

María Paz Gracia
CertVD.
Bahía de Málaga
Veterinary Referral Centre.
Parque Empresarial Laurotorre 25
Alhaurín de la Torre (Málaga, Spain).
Text and images of page 45 (c1)*, 46 (c2).

Carmen Lorente Méndez
Animal Medicine and Surgery Dep.
Faculty of Experimental and Health Sciences.
Cardenal Herrera CEU University.
Moncada (Valencia, Spain).
Text and images 39 (c1), 62 (c2).

* c1, c2 corresponds to the position of each case in the page in question, the position being numbered from left to right and top to bottom.

Foreword

This Atlas constitutes a new and valuable contribution to the literature of Veterinary Dentistry. It is not a text book; rather it uses a wide spectrum of well-organised visual material to clearly explain different oral and dental pathologies in cats.

The Spanish author has selected well-known international collaborators to contribute to a comprehensive range of high-quality visual material comprising more than 400 pictures arranged on 160 pages. The chapters and pages are laid out in a clear and interesting format that communicate information effectively and retain the reader's interest on a voyage of discovery.

The overall organisation in terms of aetiology, clinical and diagnostic features together with well-labeled diagrams and illustrations is a format that allows the reader to quickly delve down to whatever level of detail is required. In particular, the juxtaposition of different visual formats provides a multidimensional insight. For example, well-selected clinical photographs and matching radiographs highlight the value of radiography in diagnosis.

The Atlas is both a well-conceived idea and a well-executed project. This one book has such a broad coverage of oral and dental pathologies in cats that it constitutes a uniquely valuable addition to the library of any veterinary surgeon.

Cecilia Gorrel
BSc, MA, Vet MB, DDS, MRCVS, Hon FAVD, Dipl EVDC
RCVS-recognised Specialist in Veterinary Dentistry

Preface

As my interest in the field of Veterinary Dentistry and Oral Surgery started growing, I always missed having a single work where all the most frequent oral and dental pathologies would be represented visually, and was forced to immerse deeply into different books and journals in the field. I was truly eager to "see" everything that was described so well in those publications. I always wished I could have a visual work as a reference, to support the broad and excellent literature there already is in the field of Veterinary Dentistry.

In spite of that, it never occurred to me at that time that I would be entrusted with this profound and arduous task more than a decade after starting my journey in this specialisation.

I always considered that the premise "a picture is worth a thousand words" is key to the practical training of veterinary students and veterinary surgeons who have to face a clinical case in a specialty they are not completely familiar with. When I was teaching the subject of "Animal Dentistry" to senior students in Veterinary Medicine or when I was teaching training courses, I always tried to show my clinical experience in images that would stay on the recipient's retina, using high-quality images for a simple and clear identification of the oral disease. If I managed to do this with only one of my fellow colleagues, it had been worth the effort. And this is the objective of this book.

In this Atlas I have tried to include the images that best represent the pathologies in which I have specialised in. With a structure that includes clear illustrations and images of these pathologies along with diagnostic tests to highlight many of them, I hope to convey the key points to their visual identification, and guide the reader towards a precise diagnosis and treatment. I also hope this tool will be used as a quick reference for the identification and better understanding of oral and dental pathologies in cats both by general vet practitioners in their daily work and Veterinary Medicine students in their last years of the degree.

Always bearing in mind the hypothesis that "not all the listed are here but those that are here, are listed", this visual atlas is, thanks to, and especially for, the hundreds of colleagues that have left their patients to my care. It is, of course, also directed to those colleagues who have shown extraordinary and innate professionalism, devoting precious personal time to increasing their training in the specialty, with the final objective of improving the oral health of one of their patients.

I never meant to create a textbook; there is extraordinary, extensive and good-quality literature available in human and veterinary Dentistry, the latter being backed up by European and American diplomates in Veterinary Dentristry, with a truly fascinating and complete scientific content. My objective was always to gather images for a better understanding of these texts. If I fulfil my goal, I will be proud of and forever thankful to all those who have collaborated directly or directly to the creation of this work. If anyone feels disappointed, that will then be the perfect stimulus to keep growing and, from the humility of acknowledging constructive criticism, improve this work for further editions.

If only one of the 400 images stays on your retina forever, I will have far exceeded my goal and it will have been worth the effort. I hope this work will encourage you to expand your library on the speciality, as well as arouse your interest for a better training in the field of Veterinary Dentistry and Oral Surgery.

Javier Collados

Table of contents

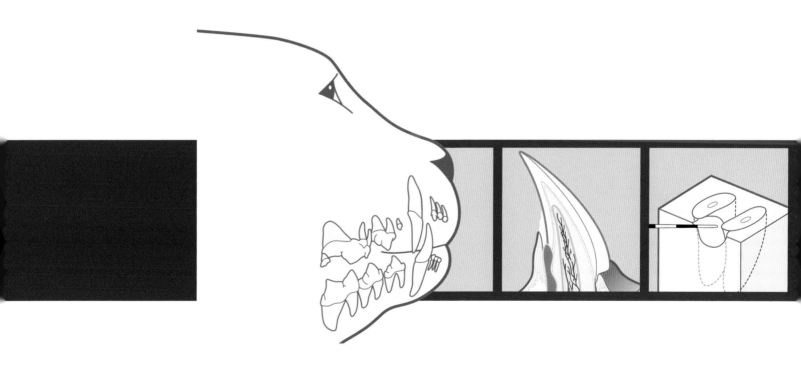

Introduction

Dental positional terminology

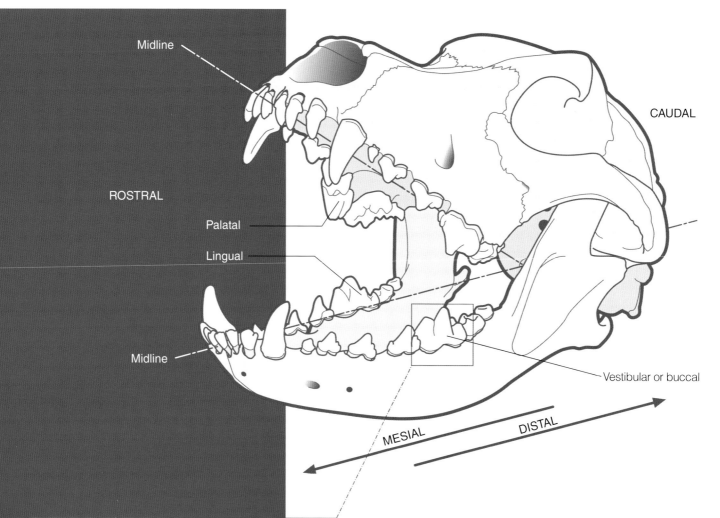

Midline

ROSTRAL

Palatal

Lingual

Midline

Vestibular or buccal

CAUDAL

MESIAL

DISTAL

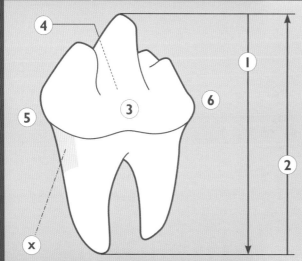

Dental positional terminology

Dental positional terminology is used to determine the location of the different surfaces and directions of each tooth or dentition:

1. **Apical:** towards the apex of the root.

2. **Coronal:** towards the crown of the tooth.

3. **Vestibular-buccal-facial-labial:** the surface of a tooth facing the vestibule or lips.

4. **Lingual (mandible)/Palatal (maxilla):** the surface of a tooth facing the tongue (mandible) or the palate (maxilla).

5. **Mesial:** the surface of a tooth towards to the first incisor.

6. **Distal:** the surface of a tooth away from the first incisor.

   Interproximal: the adjacent surfaces between teeth.

   Incisal: the biting surface of incisors.

   Occlusal: the chewing surface of the premolars and molars.

This terminology can be combined in the different dental anatomic regions to locate exact anatomical points in the tooth. For example, the area represented with the letter ⓧ is the mesial surface of the coronal third of the mesial root of the lower first molar.

Histological tooth structure in canines and felines

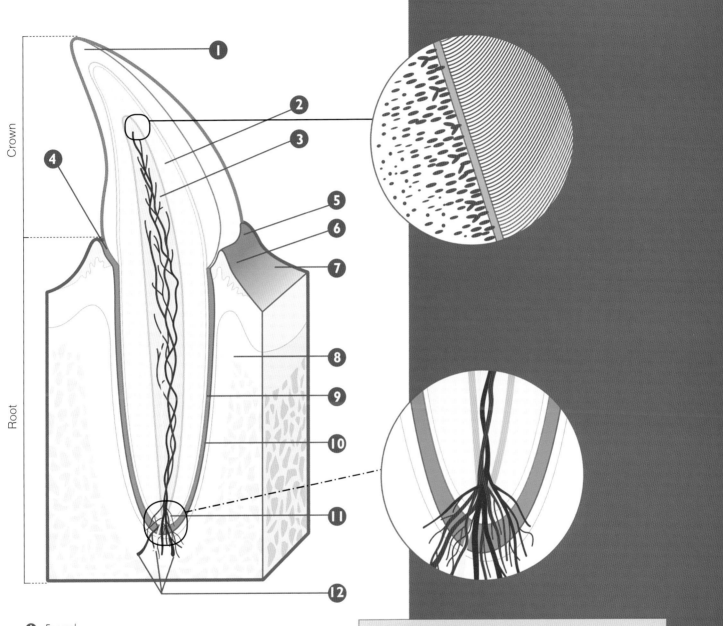

- ❶ Enamel.
- ❷ Dentin.
- ❸ Pulp cavity with dental pulp.
- ❹ Gingival sulcus.
- ❺ Free gingiva.
- ❻ Attached gingiva.
- ❼ Alveolar mucosa.
- ❽ Alveolar bone.
- ❾ Cementum.
- ❿ Periodontal ligament.
- ⓫ Apical delta.
- ⓬ Dental vascularisation and innervation.

Histological tooth structure (diagram)

The **enamel**, produced by ameloblasts, is the most mineralized surface of the organism. Dentin occupies the greater part of mature teeth in the crown-root, and is produced by odontoblasts.

Dental tubules are found in the **dentin** that are wider near the pulp and become narrower as they near the dentino-enamel junction.

The **pulp** is a vascular structure with nerve fibres, blood and lymphatic vessels and connective tissue. Dental pulp is located inside of the pulp cavity (**pulp chamber** in the crown, and **root canal** in the root).

The **periodontal ligament** is an innervated fibrous connective tissue rich in cells and vessels that possesses collagen fibres called *Sharpey's fibres*, which connect the cementum and the alveolar bone. This periodontal ligament is the structure responsible for keeping the tooth in its alveolus.

Diagram of dog and cat dentition

Nomenclature of the permanent dentition of dogs

Dog maxilla		
Right	Left	
RmaxI1 (101)	LmaxI1 (201)	a
RmaxI2 (102)	LmaxI2 (202)	b
RmaxI3 (103)	LmaxI4 (203)	c
RmaxC (104)	LmaxC (204)	d
RmaxP1 (105)	LmaxP1 (205)	e
RmaxP2 (106)	LmaxP2 (206)	f
RmaxP3 (107)	LmaxP3 (207)	g
RmaxP4 (108)	LmaxP4 (208)	h
RmaxM1 (109)	LmaxM1 (209)	i
RmaxM2 (110)	LmaxM2 (210)	j

Dog mandible		
Right	Left	
RmandI1 (401)	LmandI1 (301)	k
RmandI2 (402)	LmandI2 (302)	l
RmandI3 (403)	LmandI3 (303)	m
RmandC (404)	LmandC (304)	n
RmandP1 (405)	LmandP1 (305)	o
RmandP2 (406)	LmandP2 (306)	p
RmandP3 (407)	LmandP3 (307)	q
RmandP4 (408)	LmandP4 (308)	r
RmandM1 (409)	LmandM1 (309)	s
RmandM2 (410)	LmandM2 (310)	t
RmandM3 (411)	LmandM3 (311)	u

Dog: deciduous teeth

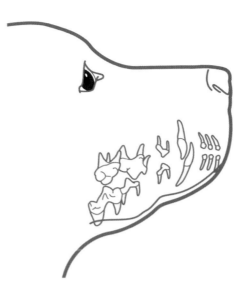

Dog: permanent teeth

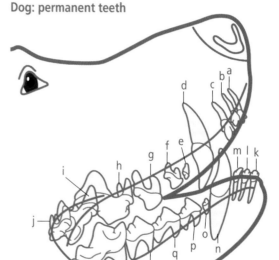

Dental nomenclature

To better understand this text, two dental nomenclatures will be used:

- **Anatomical abbreviation.** There are three parts in this system of abbreviation. In the first part, we find an abbreviation for the side on which the affected/relevant tooth is found, R (right) or L (left). In the second part, we represent if it belongs to "max" (maxilla) or to "mand" (mandible). And lastly, the third part refers to the tooth itself, represented by I (incisor), C (canine), P (premolar) or M (molar), followed by the number that corresponds with each tooth (if applicable). Following this abbreviation system, for example, RmaxP2 refers to the right upper second premolar. The exclusive use of this system is sufficient to understand this text perfectly.

Cat: deciduous teeth

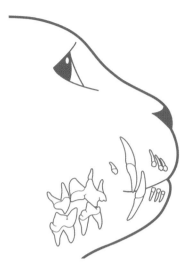

Cat: permanent teeth

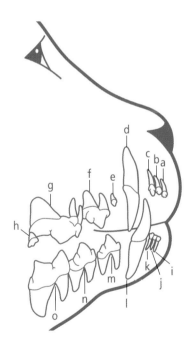

Cat maxilla		
Right	Left	
RmaxI1 (101)	LmaxI1 (201)	a
RmaxI2 (102)	LmaxI2 (202)	b
RmaxI3 (103)	LmaxI4 (203)	c
RmaxC (104)	LmaxC (204)	d
RmaxP2 (106)	LmaxP2 (206)	e
RmaxP3 (107)	LmaxP3 (207)	f
RmaxP4 (108)	LmaxP4 (208)	g
Rmax1M (109)	Lmax1M (209)	h

Cat mandible		
Right	Left	
RmandI1 (401)	LmandI1 (301)	i
RmandI2 (402)	LmandI2 (302)	j
RmandI3 (403)	LmandI3 (303)	k
RmandC (404)	LmandC (304)	l
RmandP3 (407)	LmandP3 (307)	m
RmandP4 (408)	LmandP4 (308)	n
RmandM1 (409)	LmandM1 (309)	o

■ Modified Triadan system. This system is the system of choice in veterinary Dentistry. It is a specific system of numbering and identification of teeth in human Dentistry, adapted to the anatomical differences of teeth in animals. To facilitate comprehension in this text, and for those that are familiar with this system, this nomenclature will be included in parenthesis for each tooth that is referenced using its anatomical abbreviation. For example, RmaxP2 (106).

Example of periodontal probing

In periodontal probing, the insertion of 1 to 3 mm of the periodontal probe in the gingival sulcus (depending on the species and tooth being studied) is a normal physiological finding. When we introduce the periodontal probe to a depth of 4 mm or greater, in most cases, it implies a loss of bone in that region, as well as of the periodontal ligament that was tightly attached to the tooth cementum.

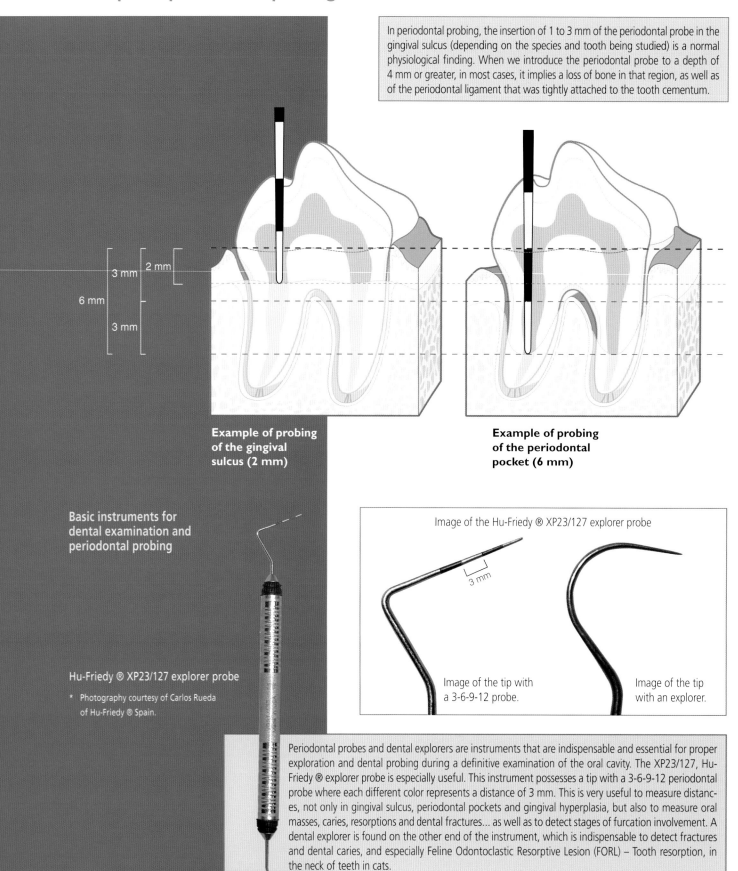

Example of probing of the gingival sulcus (2 mm)

Example of probing of the periodontal pocket (6 mm)

Basic instruments for dental examination and periodontal probing

Hu-Friedy ® XP23/127 explorer probe

* Photography courtesy of Carlos Rueda of Hu-Friedy ® Spain.

Image of the Hu-Friedy ® XP23/127 explorer probe

3 mm

Image of the tip with a 3-6-9-12 probe.

Image of the tip with an explorer.

Periodontal probes and dental explorers are instruments that are indispensable and essential for proper exploration and dental probing during a definitive examination of the oral cavity. The XP23/127, Hu-Friedy ® explorer probe is especially useful. This instrument possesses a tip with a 3-6-9-12 periodontal probe where each different color represents a distance of 3 mm. This is very useful to measure distances, not only in gingival sulcus, periodontal pockets and gingival hyperplasia, but also to measure oral masses, caries, resorptions and dental fractures... as well as to detect stages of furcation involvement. A dental explorer is found on the other end of the instrument, which is indispensable to detect fractures and dental caries, and especially Feline Odontoclastic Resorptive Lesion (FORL) – Tooth resorption, in the neck of teeth in cats.

Periodontal disease classification (AVDC, 2007)

The degree of severity of periodontal disease refers to one tooth. In the same oral cavity, different teeth may be affected by different stages of periodontal disease.

Normal. Clinically normal, no gingival inflammation or periodontitis clinically evident.

Stage 1. Gingivitis only, without attachment loss. The height and architecture of the alveolar margin are normal.

Stage 2. Early periodontitis, less than 25 % of attachment loss or at most, there is a stage 1 furcation involvement in multirooted teeth. There are early radiologic signs of periodontitis. The loss of periodontal attachment is less than 25 % as measured either by probing of the clinical attachment level, or radiographic determination of the distance of the alveolar margin from the cemento-enamel junction relative to the length of the root.

Stage 3. Moderate periodontitis, 25-50 % of attachment loss as measured either by probing of the clinical attachment level, radiographic determination of the distance of the alveolar margin from the cemento-enamel junction relative to the length of the root, or there is a stage 2 furcation involvement in multirooted teeth.

Stage 4. Advanced periodontitis, more than 50 % of attachment loss as measured either by probing of the clinical attachment level, or radiographic determination of the distance of the alveolar margin from the cemento-enamel junction relative to the length of the root, or there is a stage 3 furcation involvement in multirooted teeth.

Classification of plaque and dental calculus index (Logan & Boyce, 1994)

Plaque index (modified after Logan & Boyce, 1994)

Index 0. No plaque detected.

Index 1. 1–25 % of the crown covered by plaque.

Index 2. 25–50 % of the crown covered by plaque.

Index 3. 50–75 % of the crown covered by plaque.

Index 4. 75–100 % of the crown covered by plaque.

Calculus index (modified after Logan & Boyce, 1994)

Index 0. No calculus detected.

Index 1. 1–25 % of the crown covered by calculus.

Index 2. 25–50 % of the crown covered by calculus.

Index 3. 50–75 % of the crown covered by calculus.

Index 4. 75–100 % of the crown covered by calculus.

Gingival index
(Wolf et al., 2005)

- Index 0. Normal gingiva, no inflammation, no discoloration, no bleeding.

- Index 1. Mild inflammation, mild discoloration, mild alteration of gingival surface, no bleeding.

- Index 2. Moderate inflammation, erythema, swelling, bleeding on probing or when pressure applied.

- Index 3. Severe inflammation, severe erythema and swelling, tendency towards spontaneous bleeding, some ulceration.

Stages of mobility
(AVDC, 2007)

- Stage 0. Physiological mobility up to 0.2 mm.

- Stage 1. The mobility is increased in any direction other than axial over a distance of more than 0.2 mm and up to 0.5 mm.

- Stage 2. The mobility is increased in any direction other than axial over a distance of more than 0.5 mm and up to 1.0 mm.

- Stage 3. The mobility is increased in any direction other than axial over a distance exceeding 1.0 mm or any axial movement.

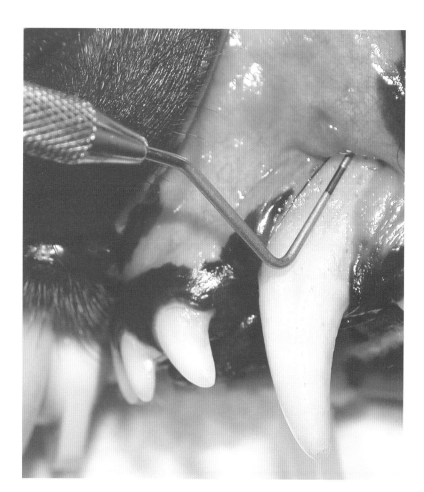

Classification of furcation involvement/exposure (AVDC, 2007)

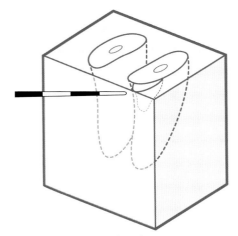

No furcation involvement

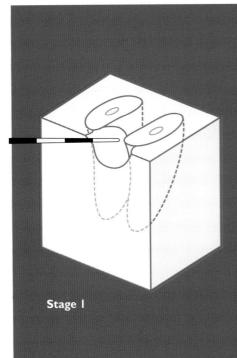

Stage 1

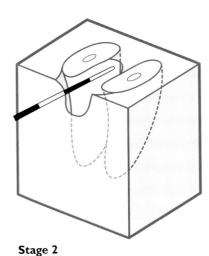

Stage 2

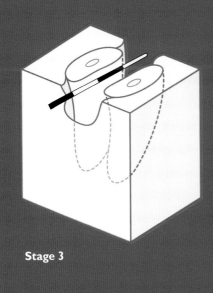

Stage 3

Stages of furcation involvement/exposure (American Veterinary Dental College, 2007).

■ Stage 0. No furcation involvement.

■ Stage 1. Furcation involvement whereby a periodontal probe extends less than half way under the crown in any direction of a multirooted tooth with attachment loss.

■ Stage 2. Furcation involvement whereby a periodontal probe extends greater than half way under the crown of a multirooted tooth with attachment loss but not through and through.

■ Stage 3. Furcation exposure whereby a periodontal probe extends under the crown of a multirooted tooth, through and through from one side of the furcation out the other.

Dental fracture classification (AVDC, 2007)

Infractions and enamel fractures have limited clinical importance, except for those causing rough surfaces that can provoke lesions in adjacent soft tissues.

Uncomplicated crown fractures are significant as exposure of the dentinal tubules can cause dental hypersensitivity.

In complicated crown fractures, pulpitis or pulp inflammation is caused by exposure of the pulp. Without adequate treatment (endodontic treatment or tooth extraction), this may lead to the appearance of pulp necrosis that will progress towards the apical delta and ultimately cause periapical pathology.

In complicated crown-root fractures, this situation will be complicated with a greater risk of periodontal disease in those areas where the fracture affects the gingival region, due to a greater deposit of bacterial plaque caused by the fracture.

Root fractures are usually candidates for tooth extraction, especially those found in the coronal third of the root. Special precaution should be taken in cats to differentiate the advanced stages of tooth resorption (very frequent pathology) with the strict root structures (less frequent and usually from traumatic or iatrogenic causes).

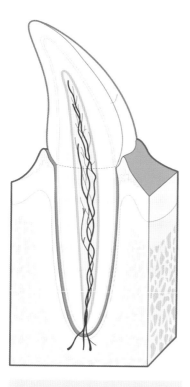

Enamel infraction: incomplete fracture ("crack") of the enamel without loss of tooth substance.

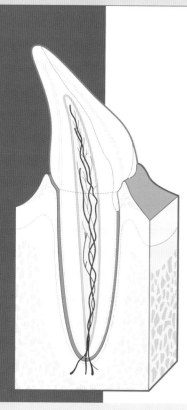

Uncomplicated crown-root fracture: fracture of the crown (enamel and dentin) and root (dentin and cementum) that does not expose the pulp.

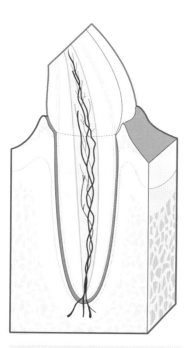

Complicated crown fracture: fracture of the crown (enamel and dentin) that exposes the pulp.

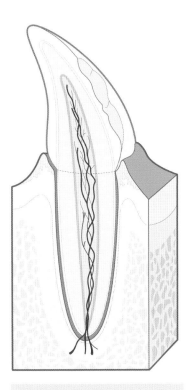

Enamel fracture: fracture with loss of crown substance confined to the enamel.

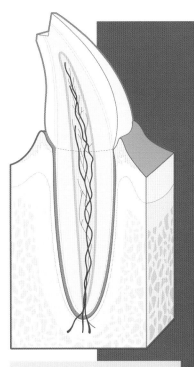

Uncomplicated crown fracture: fracture of the crown (enamel and dentin) that does not expose the pulp.

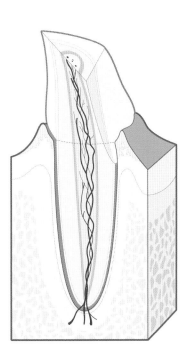

Complicated crown-root fracture: fracture of the crown (enamel and dentin) and root (dentin and cementum) that exposes the pulp.

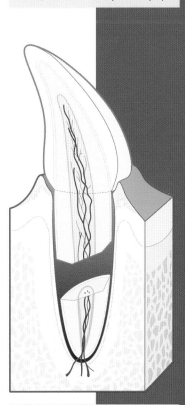

Root fracture: fracture involving the root (dentin and cementum).

Endo-periodontal lesions

Endo-periodontal lesions are of an inflammatory nature that affect, or simultaneously alter, the structures of the periodontal ligament and the dental pulp.

The classification of these lesions is based on their origin. Therefore, type I lesions are those that start as pulp lesions, where bacterial contamination that is typical of pulp necrosis migrates through the apical delta and passes through the periodontal ligament.

In type II lesions, the bacteria that are found in the deep periodontal pockets invade the pulp cavity due to its advancement through the apical delta, causing pulp necrosis.

In type III lesions, the periodontal and endodontic lesions are independent, and advance and coincide at the same time.

Type I

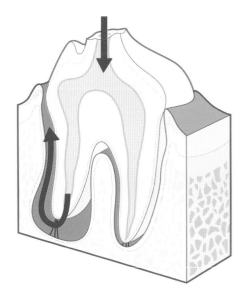

Type II

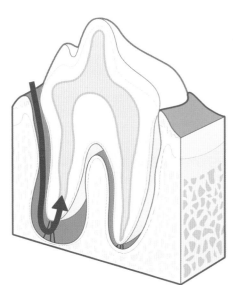

Type III

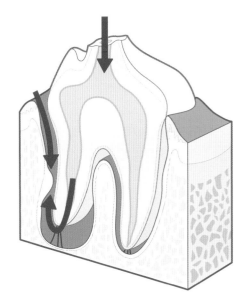

Classification of tooth resorption (based on the severity of the resorption) (AVDC, 2007)

- Stage 1. Mild dental hard tissue loss (cementum or cementum and enamel).

- Stage 2. Moderate dental hard tissue loss (cementum or cementum and enamel with loss of dentin that does not extend to the pulp cavity).

- Stage 3. Deep dental hard tissue loss (cementum or cementum and enamel with loss of dentin that extends to the pulp cavity); most of the tooth retains its integrity.

- Stage 4. Extensive deep dental hard tissue loss (cementum or cementum and enamel with loss of dentin that extends to the pulp cavity); most of the tooth loses its integrity.

  - Stage 4a. Crown and root are equally affected.

  - Stage 4b. The crown is more seriously affected than the root.

  - Stage 4c. The root is more seriously affected than the crown.

- Stage 5. Remnants of dental hard tissue are visible only as irregular radiopacities. Gingival covering is complete.

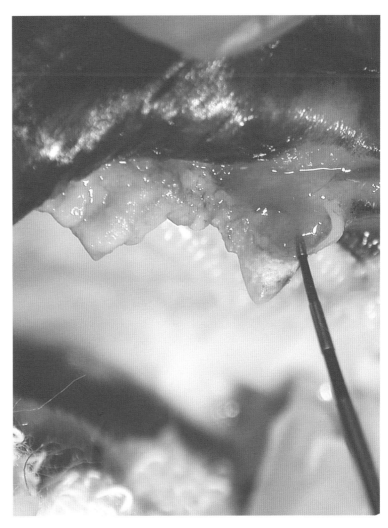

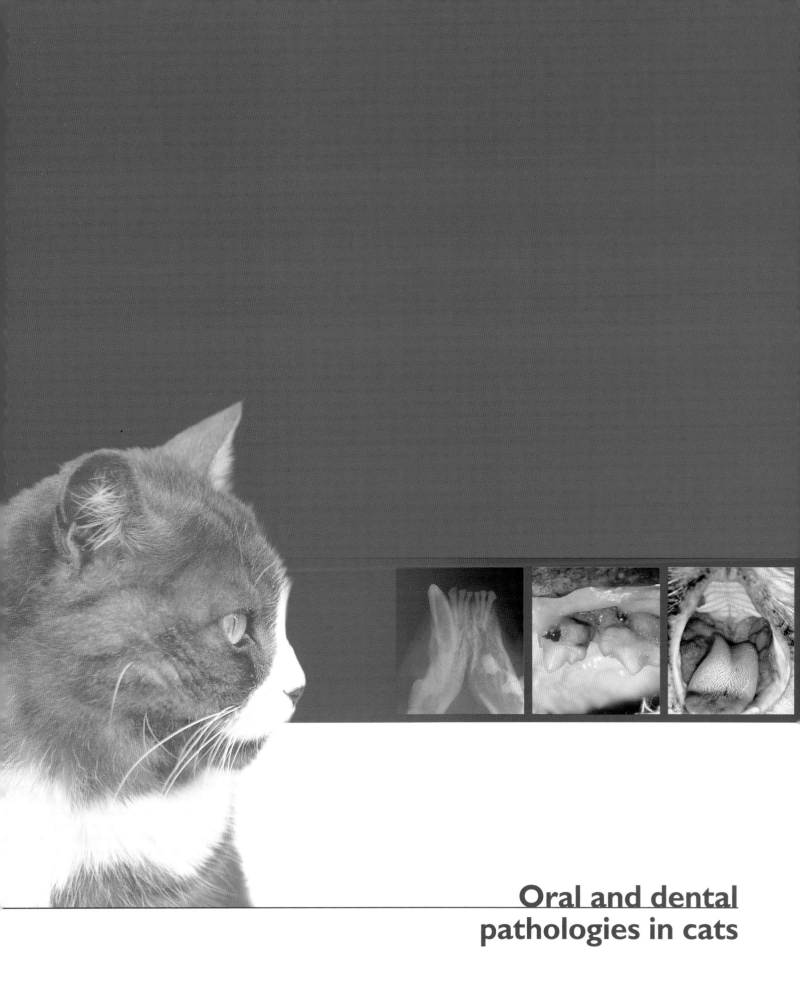

Oral and dental
pathologies in cats

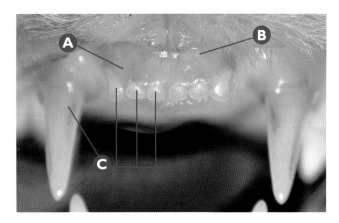
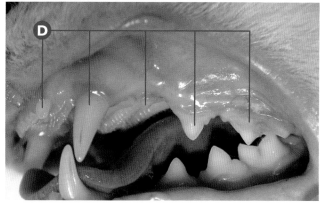
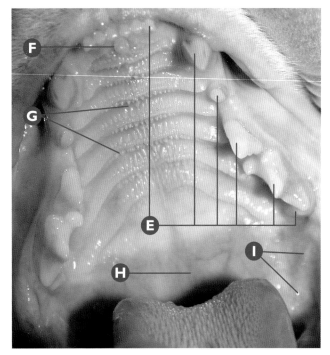
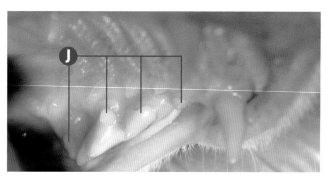
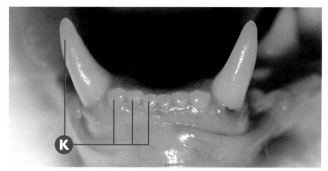

Permanent teeth

Dental anatomy and normal physiological oral cavity in cats (adults). Presence of permanent teeth.

🅐 Gingiva.

🅑 Mucosa.

🅒 From right to left: Rmaxl1 (101), Rmaxl2 (102), Rmaxl3 (103) and RmaxC (104); rostral view.

🅓 From right to left: LmaxP4 (208), LmaxP3 (207), LmaxP2 (206), LmaxC (204), LmaxI3 (203).

🅔 From right to left: LmaxM1 (209), LmaxP4 (208), LmaxP3 (207), LmaxP2 (206), LmaxC (204), LmaxI3 (203).

🅕 Incisive papilla.

🅖 Palatal ridges of the hard palate.

🅗 Soft palate.

🅘 Left caudal buccal mucosa.

🅙 From right to left: close-up of LmaxP2 (206), LmaxP3 (207), LmaxP4 (208), LmaxM1 (209).

🅚 From right to left: RmandI1 (401), RmandI2 (402), RmandI3 (403) and RmandC (404); rostral view.

🅛 From right to left: LmandM1 (309), LmandP4 (308), LmandP3 (307); vestibular view.

🅜 Labial frenulum.

🅝 Muco-gingival junction.

🅞 Feline molar gland.

🅟 From right to left: RmandM1 (409), RmandP4 (408), RmandP3 (407); lingual view.

🅠 Sublingual caruncles.

🅡 Lingual frenulum.

🅢 Left palatoglossal arch.

🅣 Papillae on the dorsal surface of the tongue.

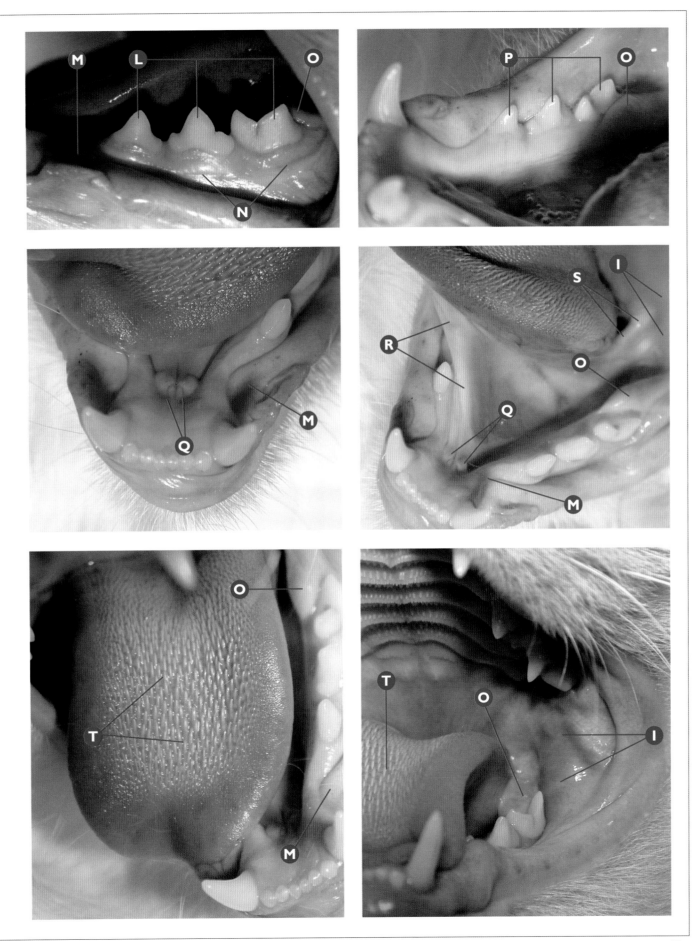

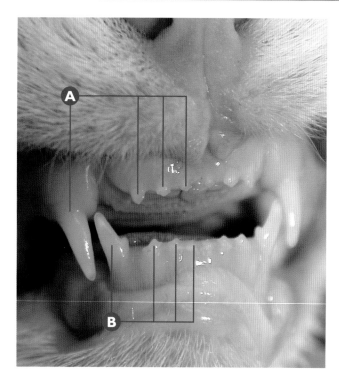
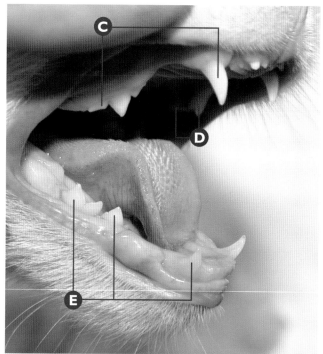

Deciduous teeth

Dental anatomy and normal physiological oral cavity in cats (kittens). Presence of deciduous teeth.

(A) From right to left, all deciduous: RmaxI1 (501), RmaxI2 (502), RmaxI3 (503) and RmaxC (504); rostral view.

(B) From right to left, all deciduous: RmandI1 (801), RmandI2 (802), RmandI3 (803) and RmandC (804); rostral view.

(C) From right to left, all deciduous: RmaxC (504) and RmaxP3 (507); vestibular view.

(D) From right to left, all deciduous: LmaxP3 (607) and LmaxP4 (608); palatal view.

(E) From right to left, all deciduous: RmandC (804), RmandP3 (807), RmandP4 (808); vestibular view.

Dental radiographic views for cats

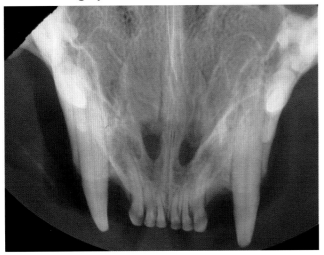

Photo 1. Intraoral occlusal view (bisecting angle technique) for radiological assessment of the incisor and canine teeth in the maxilla, in a 6-year-old patient.

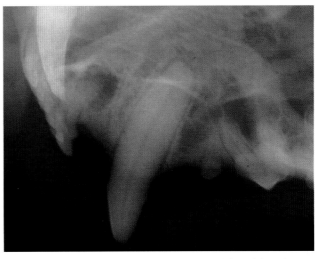

Photo 2. Intraoral lateral view (bisecting angle technique) for radiological assessment of the left maxillary canine tooth (LmaxC), in a 6-year-old patient.

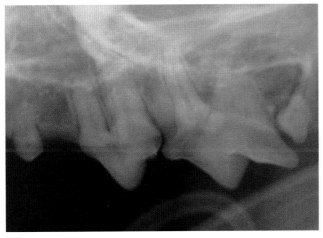

Photo 3. Extraoral view of the left maxilla (parallel technique with a slightly modified angle) for radiological assessment of the premolars and molar (LmaxP2, LmaxP3, LmaxP4, LmaxM1) in a 6-year-old patient.

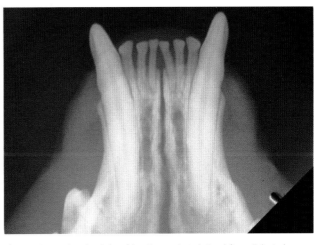

Photo 4. Intraoral occlusal view (bisecting angle technique) for radiological assessment of the mandibular incisor and canine teeth, in a 6-year-old patient.

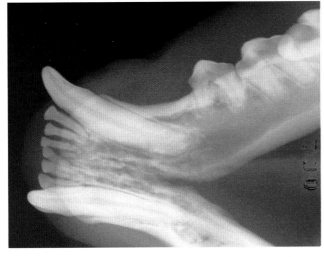

Photo 5. Intraoral lateral view (bisecting angle technique) for radiological assessment of the left mandibular canine tooth (LmandC), in a 6-year-old patient.

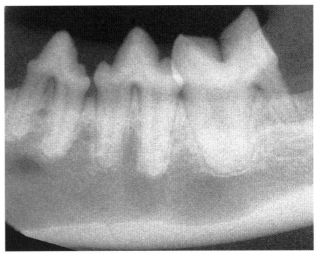

Photo 6. Intraoral view of the left mandible (parallel technique) for radiological assessment of the premolars and molar (LmandP3, LmandP4, LmandM1) in a 6-year-old patient.

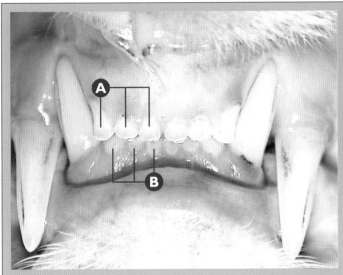

Occlusion | Incisor area

Normal physiological occlusion in the incisor area (permanent teeth).

Ⓐ From right to left: RmaxI1 (101), RmaxI2 (102), RmaxI3 (103).

Ⓑ From right to left: RmandI1 (401), RmandI2 (402), RmandI3 (403).

Key diagnostic/treatment points
The occlusion in the incisor area in this case is a physiological occlusion in numerous breeds.

The cusp of each lower incisor occludes on the distal surface of the crown of its upper counterpart.

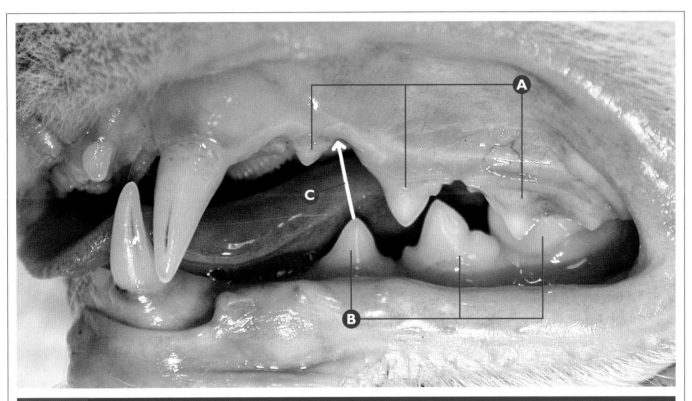

Occlusion | Premolar and molar area

Normal physiological occlusion in the premolar and molar area (permanent teeth).

Ⓐ From right to left: LmaxP4 (208), LmaxP3 (207), LmaxP2 (206); incomplete occlusion for visualisation of LmandM1 (309).

Ⓑ From right to left: LmandM1 (309), LmandP4 (308), LmandP3 (307).

Ⓒ The cusp of LmandP3 (307) will "point" towards the mesial interdental space of LmaxP3 (207) upon complete closure of the oral cavity.

Key diagnostic/treatment points
In normal physiological occlusion (incomplete in this case for visualisation of LmandM1), the cusp of each lower premolar is directed towards the mesial interdental space of its upper counterpart; for example, the cusp of LmandP3 (307) "points" towards the mesial interdental space of LmaxP3 (207). LmandM1 (309) occludes in the palatal area of LmaxP4 (208).

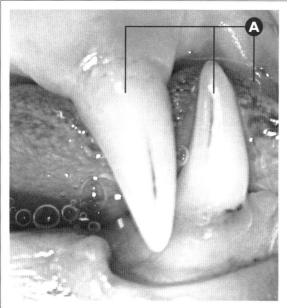
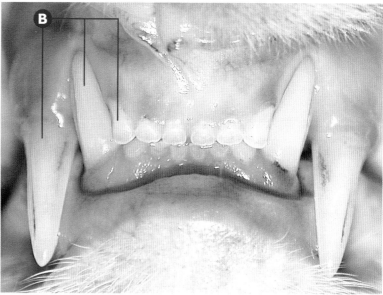

Occlusion | **Canine area**

Normal physiological occlusion in the canine area (permanent teeth).

Ⓐ From right to left: RmaxI3 (103), RmandC (404) and RmaxC (104); vestibular view.

Ⓑ From right to left: RmaxI3 (103), RmandC (404) and RmaxC (104); rostral view.

Key diagnostic/treatment points
In the normal occlusion of the canine teeth, the lower canine tooth should be located at an equal distance between the third incisor tooth and the upper canine counterpart.

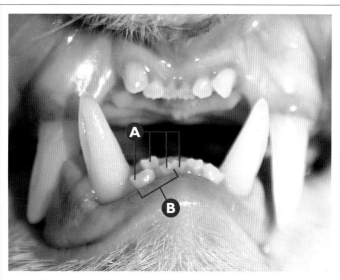
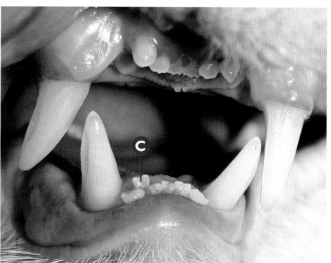

Malocclusion | **Dental crowding**

Dental crowding of the lower incisor teeth.

Ⓐ From right to left: LmandI1 (301), RmandI1 (401), RmandI2 (402), RmandI3 (403).

Ⓑ Dental crowding of RmandI1 (401), RmandI2 (402), RmandI3 (403), with distoversion (distal deviation) of RmandI2 (402).

Ⓒ Close-up of the distoversion of RmandI2 (402).

Key diagnostic/treatment points
Detection of dental crowding in the lower incisor teeth is rare in cats. It is usually found in cases where the distance between the lower canine teeth is reduced. This condition predisposes to regional periodontal disease.

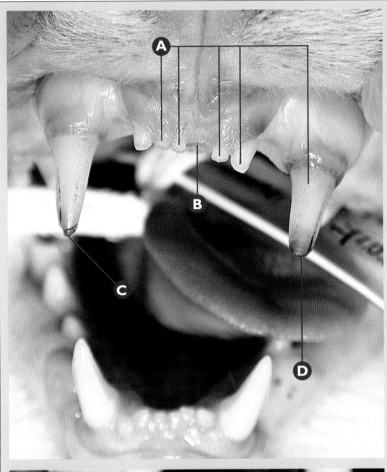

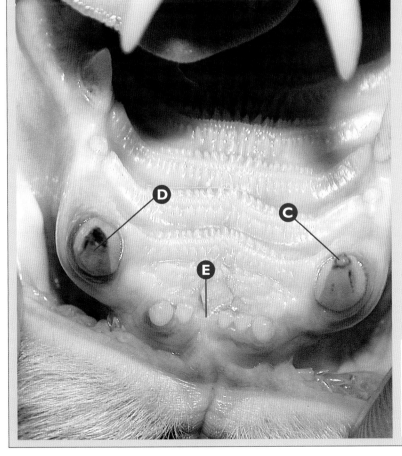

Absence of LmaxI1 (201).

Ⓐ From right to left: LmaxC (204), LmaxI3 (203), LmaxI2 (202), RmaxI1 (101), RmaxI2 (102).

Ⓑ Absence of LmaxI1 (201).

Ⓒ Suspicions of an enamel fracture of RmaxC (104).

Ⓓ Suspicions of a complicated crown fracture of LmaxC (204).

Ⓔ Close-up of the absence of LmaxI1 (201).

Key diagnostic/treatment points

In this clinical case, we can observe the absence of LmaxI1 (201), with a wide range of possible causes, from dental agenesis to dental extraction, a root fracture, advanced stage of tooth resorption or periodontal disease, etc. Dental X-rays will provide more information about the possible aetiology.

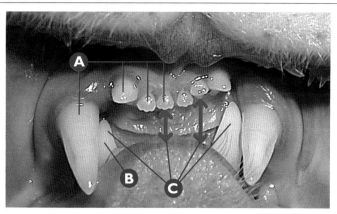
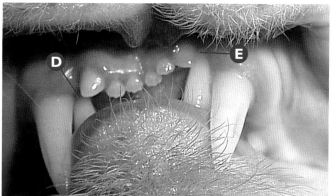

Malocclusion | **Mandibular distocclusion (class 2 malocclusion)**

Suspicions of severe mandibular distocclusion in a 10-month-old Persian cat (incisor and canine areas).

Ⓐ From right to left: RmaxI1 (101), RmaxI2 (102), RmaxI3 (103) and RmaxC (104).

Ⓑ RmandC (404).

Ⓒ Suspicions of severe mandibular distocclusion, with malocclusion of the lower incisor and canine teeth.

Ⓓ Image of the malocclusion of RmandC (404) in the palatal area of RmaxC (104).

Ⓔ Image of the malocclusion of LmandC (304) in the mesiopalatal area of LmaxC (204).

Key diagnostic/treatment points

Whenever there are suspicions of mandibular distocclusion, the occlusion of the premolars and molars must be assessed, although this region is more difficult to evaluate in cats than in dogs. In this clinical case, and especially since the patient is of the Persian breed, the suspicions are highly likely to be confirmed. The greatest complications that can be observed in this clinical case are the consequences of the dental malocclusions, especially of the canine teeth; the lower canine teeth cause impingement of the palate in different regions and cause lesions that must be assessed.

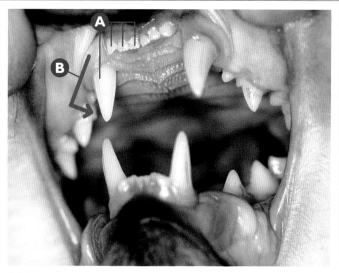
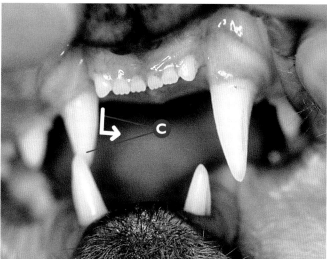

Malocclusion | **Maxillomandibular asymmetry (class 4 malocclusion)**

Suspicions of maxillomandibular asymmetry in a rostrocaudal direction (incisor and canine area).

Ⓐ From right to left: RmaxI1 (101), RmaxI2 (102), RmaxI3 (103), RmaxC (104).

Ⓑ Suspicions of severe maxillomandibular asymmetry in a rostrocaudal direction, which is more severe and noticeable on the right side.

Ⓒ Close-up of the distal and palatal position of RmaxC (104), due to maxillomandibular asymmetry in a rostrocaudal direction.

Key diagnostic/treatment points

Suspicions of severe maxillomandibular asymmetry in a rostrocaudal direction require the assessment of the occlusion of the premolars in the distal region and of the molars. In this clinical case, the maxillomandibular asymmetry in a rostrocaudal direction is more noticeable on the right side, with the resulting malocclusion.

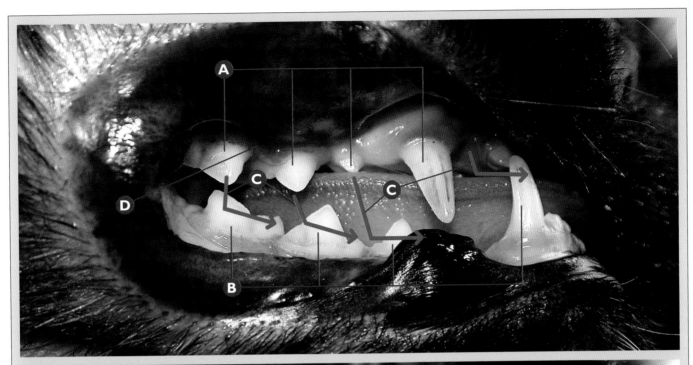

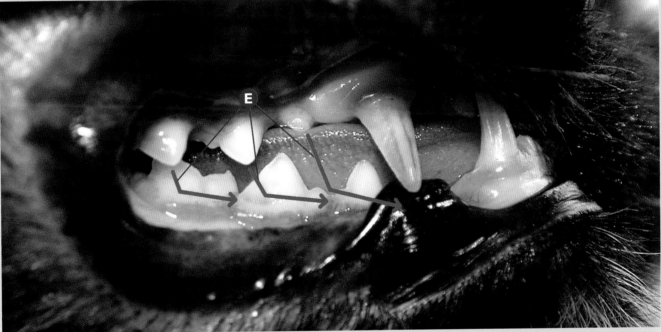

Malocclusion | **Mandibular mesiocclusion (class 3 malocclusion)**

Suspicions of severe mandibular mesiocclusion (in the area of the canine and premolars/molars on the right side).

Ⓐ From right to left: RmaxC (104), RmaxP2 (106), RmaxP3 (107) and RmaxP4 (108).

Ⓑ From right to left: RmandC (404), RmandP3 (407), RmandP4 (408) and RmandM1 (409).

Ⓒ Suspicions of severe mandibular mesiocclusion due to malocclusion in the area of the canine and premolar teeth.

Ⓓ Crowding of RmaxP3 (107) and RmaxP4 (108), which confirms the suspicions of mandibular mesiocclusion.

Ⓔ Image of the suspected severe mandibular mesiocclusion, in the area of the premolars and molars.

Key diagnostic/treatment points
The suspicions of severe mandibular mesiocclusion in this clinical case are based on the occlusion of the canine teeth and premolars/molars. RmandC (404) occludes in an extremely mesial direction compared to its location in normal occlusion. Similarly, the malocclusion has distally displaced the physiological occlusion of the upper premolars on the right side of the oral cavity.

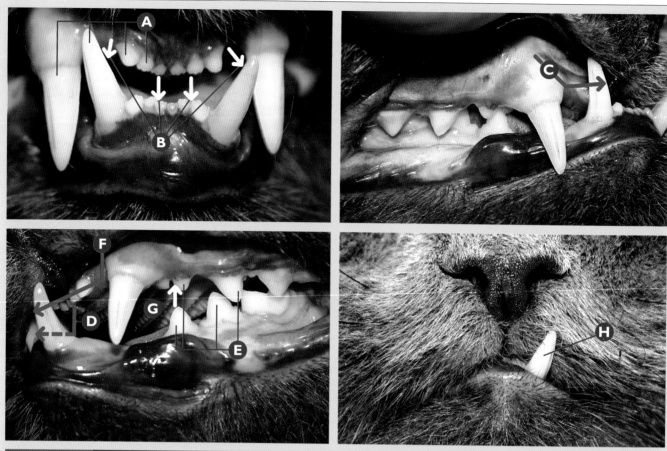

| Malocclusion | Mandibular mesiocclusion (class 3 malocclusion) |

Severe mandibular mesiocclusion (area of the canine teeth and premolars/molars on the right and left sides).

Ⓐ From right to left: RmaxI2 (102), RmaxI3 (103), RmandC (404) and RmaxC (104).

Ⓑ Suspicions of mandibular mesiocclusion due to malocclusion in the area of the incisor and canine teeth.

Ⓒ Severe mandibular mesiocclusion, due to occlusion in an extremely mesial direction of RmandC (404); right vestibular view.

Ⓓ Occlusion of the upper incisors in the area distal to the lower incisor teeth; left vestibular view.

Ⓔ From right to left: LmaxP3 (207), LmandP4 (308), LmaxP2 (206) and LmandP3 (307); left vestibular view.

Ⓕ Malocclusion of LmandC (304) in an extremely mesial direction; left vestibular view.

Ⓖ The cusp of LmandP3 (307) "points" towards the mesial area of LmaxP2 (206); left vestibular view.

Ⓗ Malocclusion of LmandC (304), outside of the oral cavity due to severe mandibular prognathism, more marked in the left mandible.

Key diagnostic/treatment points

The severe mandibular mesiocclusion in this clinical case is caused by a malocclusion of the incisor and canine teeth and premolars/molars on both sides. In the physiological occlusion, the cusp of the lower canine teeth occludes between the third incisor tooth and the upper canine tooth. However, these occlude in an extremely mesial direction compared to their location in normal physiological occlusion. Likewise, the mandibular mesiocclusion has displaced the occlusion of the lower premolars and molars in a mesial direction.

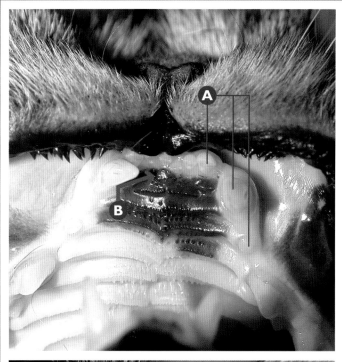

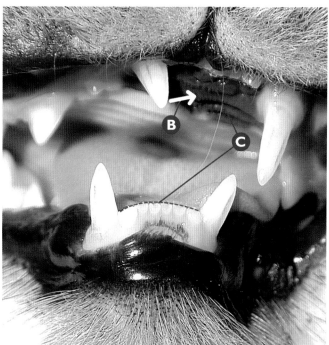

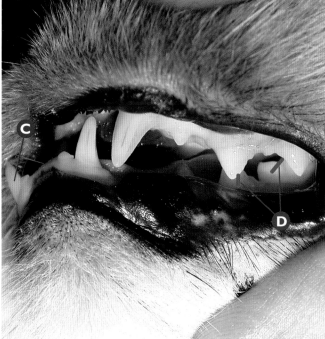

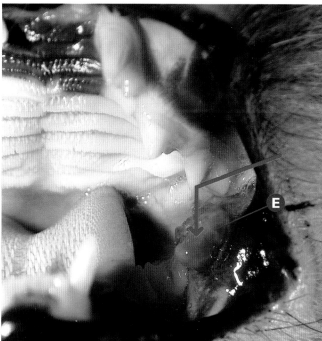

Malocclusion | **Dental deviation**

Mesiopalatal deviation of RmaxC (104).

Ⓐ From right to left: LmaxP2 (206), LmaxC (204) and LmaxI3 (203).

Ⓑ Mesiopalatal deviation of RmaxC (104).

Ⓒ Suspicions of maxillomandibular asymmetry in a side-to-side direction.

Ⓓ Space increase in the areas of contact when occluding on the premolars and molars on the left side; the most probable aetiology is maxillomandibular asymmetry in a side-to-side direction.

Ⓔ Formation of granulation tissue due to malocclusion of LmaxP4 (208) over the vestibular mucosa; the most probable aetiology is maxillomandibular asymmetry in a side-to-side direction.

Key diagnostic/treatment points
In this clinical case, there is displacement relative to the transverse axis of RmaxC (104), resulting in mesial and palatal deviation. The assessment of the occlusion is significantly interfered with as the process is combined with suspicions of maxillomandibular asymmetry in a side-to-side direction.

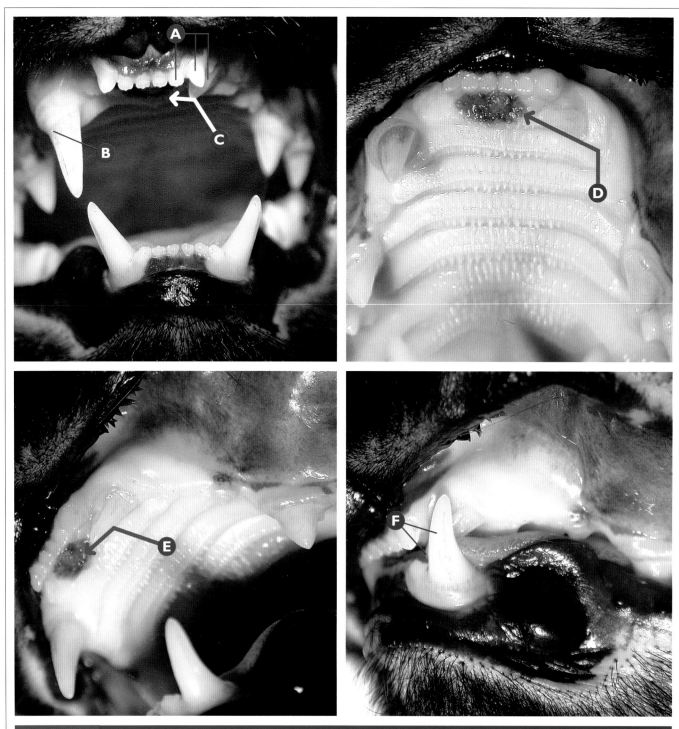

| Malocclusion | Dental deviation |

Mesiopalatal deviation of LmaxC (204).

Ⓐ From right to left: LmaxC (204), LmaxI3 (203) and LmaxI2 (202).

Ⓑ Calculus index 2 on RmaxC (104).

Ⓒ Mesiopalatal deviation of LmaxC (204); rostral view.

Ⓓ Image of the mesiopalatal deviation of LmaxC (204); intraoral view.

Ⓔ Image of the mesiopalatal deviation of LmaxC (204); rostral-vestibular view.

Ⓕ Image of the malocclusion of LmaxC (204), with the vestibular surface of the coronal third of the crown of this tooth coming into contact with the lingual surface of LmandC (304).

Key diagnostic/treatment points

In this clinical case, there is also displacement relative to the transverse axis of LmaxC (204), resulting in mesiopalatal deviation of the tooth. Occasionally, the cusp of the affected tooth bites into the soft tissues and the lower teeth, making treatment necessary to avoid this.

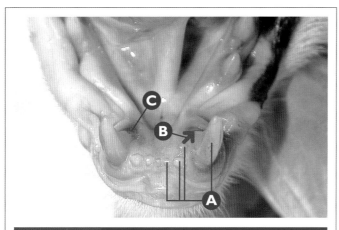

Malocclusion   Distal deviation

Distal deviation of LmandI2 (302).

Ⓐ From right to left: LmandC (304), LmandI2 (302), LmandI3 (303) and LmandI1 (301).

Ⓑ Distal deviation of LmandI2 (302).

Ⓒ Moderate gingival recession in the distolingual area of RmandC (404).

Key diagnostic/treatment points
In clinical cases where there is no physical space for proper dental eruption, rotations or deviations such as that seen here may occur. The most probable aetiology of the distal deviation of LmandI2 (302) is the modification of the direction of the dental eruption due to a lack of space between LmandI1 (301) and LmandI3 (303).

Malocclusion   Dental deviation

Mesiopalatal deviation of LmaxC (204).

Ⓐ Mesiopalatal deviation of LmaxC (204); vestibular view.

Ⓑ From right to left: LmaxC (204), LmaxI3 (203), LmaxI2 (202), LmaxI1 (201), and RmaxC (104).

Ⓒ Image of the mesiopalatal deviation of LmaxC (204); rostral view.

Ⓓ Calculus index 2 on RmaxC (104).

Ⓔ From right to left: image of the normal physiological occlusion of RmandC (404) and RmaxC (104).

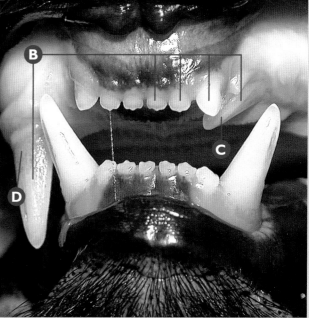

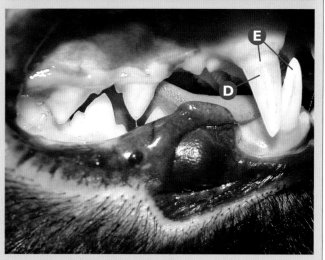

Key diagnostic/treatment points
Mesial deviation of the upper permanent canine teeth is relatively frequent, especially in the Persian breed. In this clinical case, the malocclusion detected, a mesiopalatal deviation of LmaxC (204), does not cause any modifications to the surrounding soft tissues. However, both conservative treatment (orthodontic) and non-conservative treatment (extraction) should be offered (after performing a complete dental radiological study) to the client to prevent oral disease in this area, such as periodontal disease.

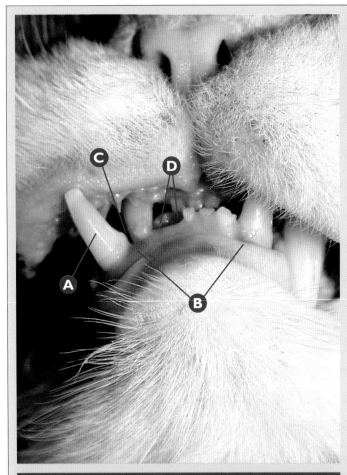

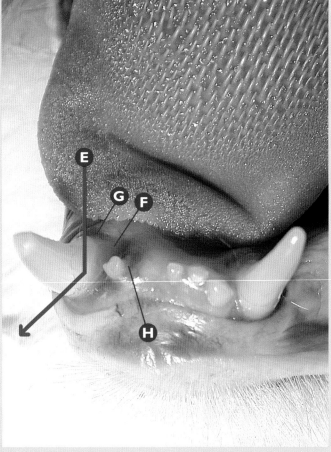

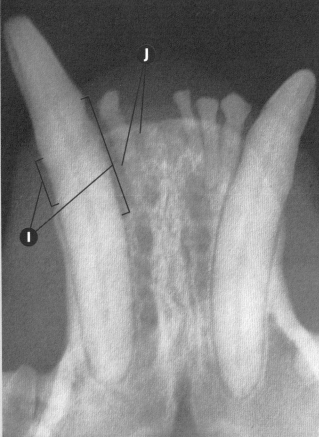

Malocclusion | Dental deviation

Vestibular deviation of RmandC (404) due to malocclusion of RmaxC (101), in a case of moderate mandibular mesiocclusion.

Ⓐ RmandC (404).

Ⓑ Moderate mandibular prognathism.

Ⓒ RmaxC (101) occluding on the distal area of RmandC (404).

Ⓓ From right to left: absence of RmandI1 (401) and RmandI2 (402).

Ⓔ Vestibular deviation of RmandC (404).

Ⓕ Contact area of the cusp of RmaxC (101) in the lingual area of RmandC (404).

Ⓖ Suspicions of stage 3 periodontal disease in RmandC (404).

Ⓗ Suspicions of stage 4 periodontal disease in RmandI3 (403).

Ⓘ Dental X-ray: radiological signs compatible with stage 3 periodontal disease in RmandC (404).

Ⓙ Dental X-ray: radiological signs compatible with stage 4 periodontal disease in RmandI3 (403).

Key diagnostic/treatment points

In this case of mandibular mesiocclusion in a Persian cat, there is malocclusion of RmaxC (101), occluding on and causing constant trauma to the lingual area of RmandC (404), thus producing a vestibular deviation of the tooth. This process favours the progress of periodontal disease in this tooth.

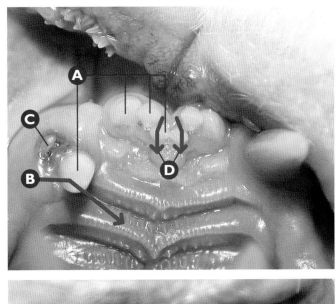

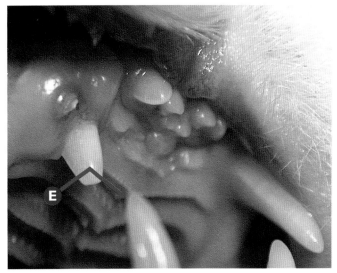

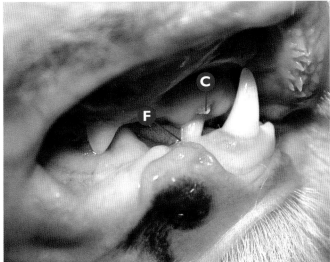

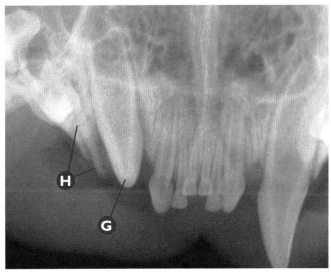

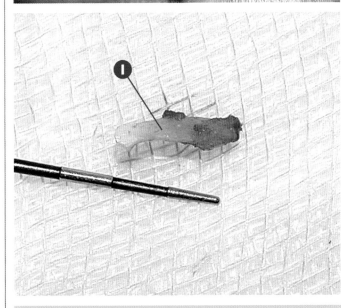

Malocclusion — Dental deviation

Distopalatal deviation of RmaxC (104), due to the presence of a root fragment of the deciduous RmaxC (504).

A From right to left: RmaxI1 (101), RmaxI2 (102), RmaxI3 (103), RmaxC (104).

B Distopalatal deviation of RmaxC (104).

C Suspicions of a root fragment of the deciduous RmaxC (504).

D Palatal deviation of RmaxI1 (101) and LmaxI1 (201).

E Close-up of the distopalatal deviation and absence of complete eruption of RmaxC (104).

F Cusp of RmaxC (104) causing impingement of the mucosa of the distal area of RmandC (404), due to its deviation.

G Dental X-ray: radiological signs compatible with RmaxC (104).

H Dental X-ray: radiological signs compatible with a root fragment of the deciduous RmaxC (504).

I Close-up of the root fragment of the deciduous RmaxC (504), after its extraction.

Key diagnostic/treatment points

Persistent teeth, along with fragments of their roots as shown in this clinical case, may cause the deviation of permanent teeth due to the interference in their normal and adequate eruption. Interceptive orthodontics should be performed when faced with a persistent tooth, that is, any persisting deciduous teeth should be extracted. Regional dental X-rays are indispensable to assess the presence, shape, partial resorption, etc. of the deciduous teeth.

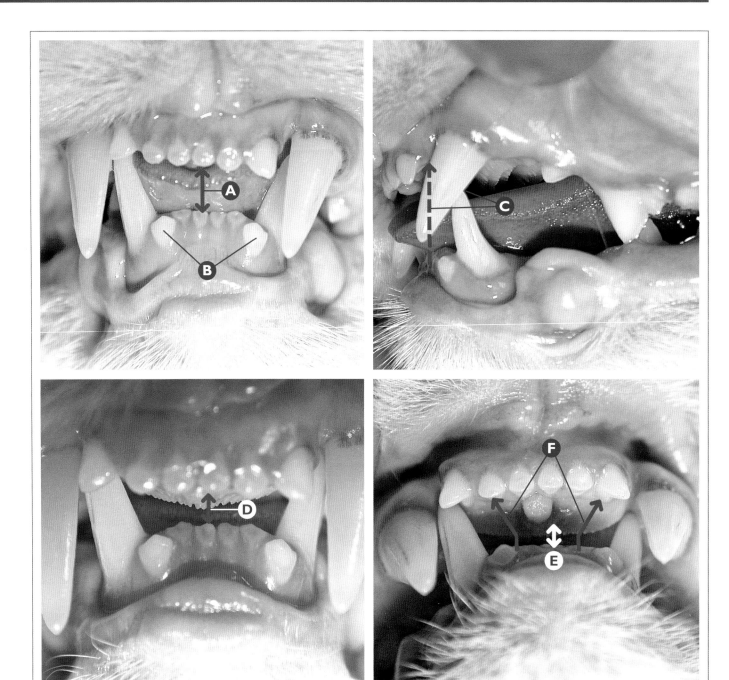

Malocclusion | **Open bite**

Severe open bite due to mandibular distocclusion (class 2 malocclusion).

Ⓐ Inability to completely close the oral cavity due to malocclusion.

Ⓑ From right to left: Vestibular deviation of LmandI3 (303) and RmandI3 (403).

Ⓒ Suspicions of severe mandibular distocclusion, with malocclusion of the lower incisor and canine teeth.

Ⓓ Inability to completely close the oral cavity; forced occlusion under sedation; rostral view.

Ⓔ Image of the inability to completely close the oral cavity; forced occlusion under sedation.

Ⓕ Image of the suspected mandibular distocclusion.

Key diagnostic/treatment points
An open bite is any malocclusion that, due to dental or skeletal discrepancy, impedes the closure of the oral cavity. In this clinical case, mandibular distocclusion (skeletal malocclusion) is the cause of the inability to close the oral cavity, even when forcing closure with the animal under sedation.

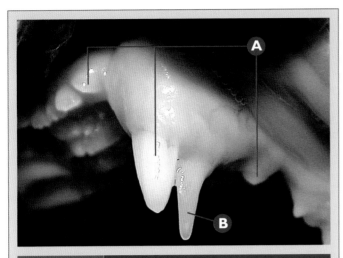

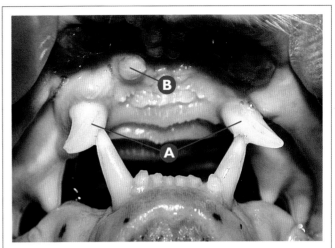

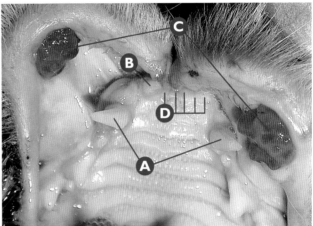

Malocclusion | Persistent tooth

Persistence of the deciduous LmaxC (604).

Ⓐ From right to left: LmaxP2 (206), LmaxC (204) and LmaxI3 (203).

Ⓑ Deciduous LmaxC (604).

Key diagnostic/treatment points
A persistent tooth is any deciduous tooth that has not been lost during exfoliation. The joint existence of a deciduous tooth and its permanent counterpart may cause secondary malocclusions, making interceptive orthodontics (extraction of the persistent tooth) highly recommended. This malocclusion is uncommon in cats.

Malocclusion | Dental rotation

Vestibular rotation of the distal area of RmaxC (104) and LmaxC (204).

Ⓐ From right to left: vestibular rotation of LmaxC (204) and RmaxC (104).

Ⓑ RmaxI3 (103).

Ⓒ Granulomatous lesions caused by the cusps of both upper canine teeth, due to the rotation.

Ⓓ From right to left: image of LmaxI3 (203), LmaxI2 (202), LmaxI1 (201), RmaxI1 (101) and RmaxI2 (102).

Ⓔ Dental X-ray: radiological signs compatible with endodontic disease due to asymmetry of the diameter of the pulp chambers.

Ⓕ Dental X-ray: radiological signs compatible with tooth resorption in the upper incisor teeth.

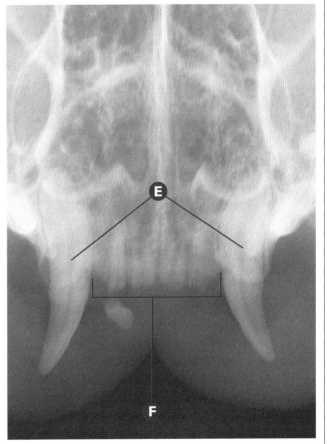

Key diagnostic/treatment points
This atypical rotation in the upper canine teeth is likely of congenital aetiology, and causes malocclusion and consequent damage to the mucosa that comes into contact with the cusps.

33

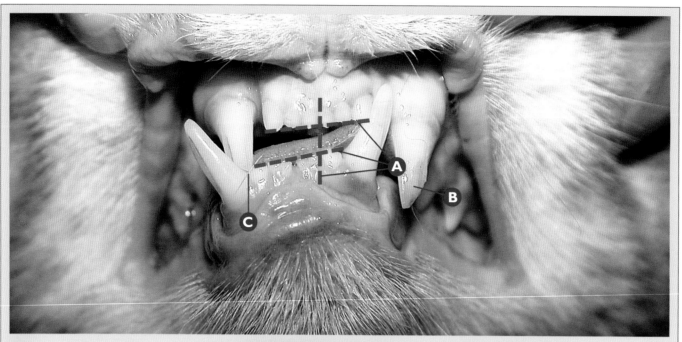

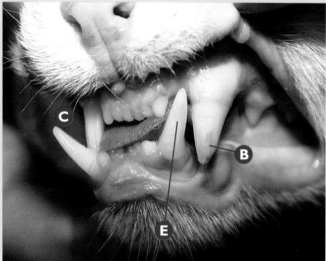

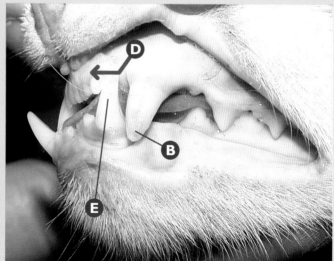

Malocclusion | **Maxillomandibular asymmetry in a side-to-side direction**

Acquired maxillomandibular asymmetry in a dorsoventral direction due to a previous trauma; inadequate spontaneous resolution of a mandibular fracture.

Ⓐ Midline deviation between the upper and lower incisor teeth, as well as asymmetry of the incisal plane; deviation towards the right side.

Ⓑ Suspicions of a complicated crown fracture of LmaxC (204).

Ⓒ Malocclusion of RmaxC (104), with its cusp occluding on the distal area of RmandC (404).

Ⓓ Mesial displacement of LmandC (304), due to the acquired maxillomandibular asymmetry in a dorsoventral direction.

Ⓔ Suspicions of an enamel fracture of the crown of LmandC (304).

Key diagnostic/treatment points
Like with dogs, this midline deviation or maxillomandibular asymmetry in a dorsoventral direction may have a congenital or acquired origin. Congenital cases (generally considered to have a genetic aetiology) may have their origin in the skeletal and dental base, or only in the dental base. In this clinical case, the aetiology of the process is acquired; in those cases in which mandibular and/or maxillary fractures are not adequately resolved, or they are spontaneously resolved in a non-physiological occlusion, malocclusions may take place.

Common errors
In cases of maxillary/mandibular trauma, whether there is visible damage or not (which would require surgical resolution), a common error is to not evaluate the patient's resulting occlusion closely and precisely (especially in the area of the canine teeth). We must focus all our efforts on reestablishing a normal physiological occlusion.

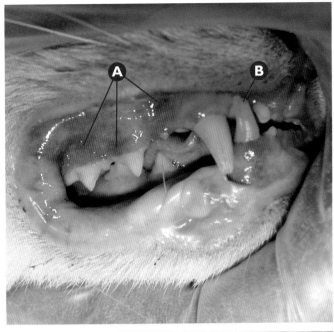
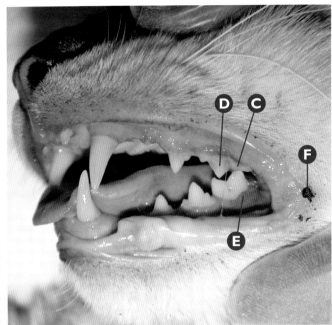
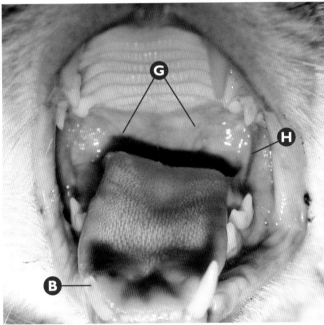
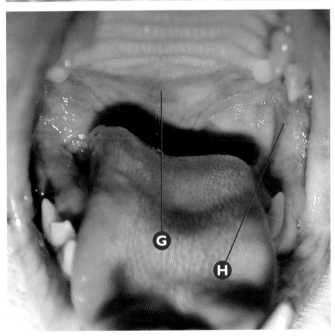

Leukaemia and feline immunodeficiency (FeLV, FIV)

Mild to moderate stomatitis due to leukaemia (FeLV) and feline immunodeficiency (FIV) in a 2-year-old patient; combined with feline calicivirus (FCV) and under antibiotic treatment. Viral analysis (PCR): **FeLV +, FIV +, FCV +, FHV -.**

Ⓐ Moderate stomatitis in the regional mucosa of RmaxP2 (106), RmaxP3 (107) and RmaxP4 (108).

Ⓑ Suspicions of a complicated crown fracture of RmandC (404).

Ⓒ Plaque index 2 on LmaxP4 (208).

Ⓓ Calculus index 2 on LmaxP4 (208).

Ⓔ Gingival index 2 in LmandM1 (309).

Ⓕ Small ulcer in the labial commissure.

Ⓖ Mild stomatitis in the soft palate.

Ⓗ Mild stomatitis in the left caudal buccal mucosa.

Key diagnostic/treatment points

Leukaemia and feline immunodeficiency are caused by two viruses of the *Retroviridae* family. Although the most important clinical signs of both diseases are systemic, lesions in the oral cavity, such as different degrees of gingivostomatitis, are often observed. The diagnosis and systemic treatment of both diseases, together with the control of the side effects, is fundamental to improve the oral and behavioural clinical signs.

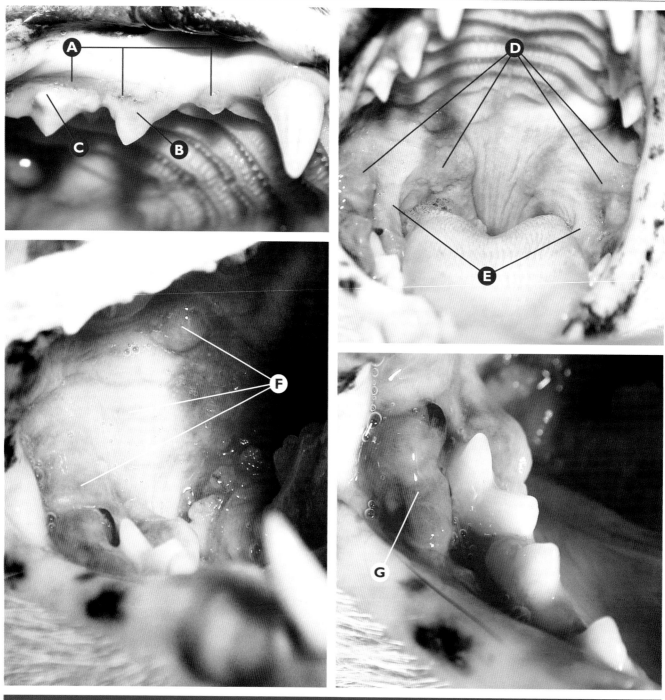

Leukaemia and feline immunodeficiency (FeLV, FIV)

Moderate gingivostomatitis due to leukaemia (FeLV) and calicivirus (FCV) in an 8-year-old patient. Viral analysis (PCR): **FeLV +, FIV -, FCV +, FHV -.**

A From right to left: gingival index 1 in RmaxP2 (106), RmaxP3 (107) and RmaxP4 (108).

B Calculus index 2 on RmaxP3 (107).

C Calculus index 1 on RmaxP4 (108).

D Moderate stomatitis in the caudal buccal mucosa on the right and left sides.

E Lesions in the palatoglossal arch due to mild/moderate stomatitis.

F Close-up of the moderate stomatitis in the right caudal buccal mucosa.

G Suspicions of hyperplastic tissue in the vestibular area of RmandM1 (409), typical in many cases of chronic feline gingivostomatitis.

Key diagnostic/treatment points

In this clinical case, leukaemia (FeLV) and feline calicivirus (FCV) are the most probable causes of the gingivostomatitis observed, although the presence of periodontal disease may worsen the clinical signs. The correct diagnosis of the underlying pathologies will help identify possible treatments and, above all, determine the general prognosis of the process.

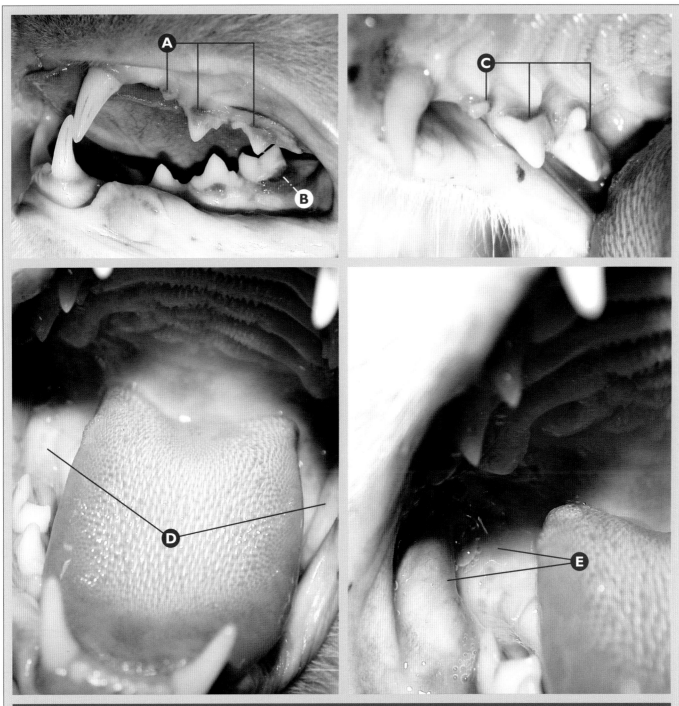

Leukaemia and feline immunodeficiency (FeLV, FIV)

Mild-moderate gingivostomatitis with presence of leukaemia (FeLV) and calicivirus (FCV) in an 18-month-old patient.
Viral analysis (PCR): FeLV +, FIV -, FCV +, FHV -.

Ⓐ From right to left: gingival index 1 in LmaxP4 (208), LmaxP3 (207) and LmaxP2 (206).

Ⓑ Gingival index 3 in LmandM1 (309).

Ⓒ From right to left: gingival index 1 in the palatal area of RmaxP4 (108), RmaxP3 (107) and RmaxP4 (106).

Ⓓ Absence of stomatitis in the caudal buccal mucosa on the right and left sides.

Ⓔ Close-up of the absence of stomatitis in the caudal buccal mucosa on the right side.

Key diagnostic/treatment points

In this clinical case, we can observe the presence of gingivitis, most likely related to the periodontal disease. Although leukaemia (FeLV) and calicivirus (FCV) were detected by PCR, no signs of gingivostomatitis in the caudal buccal mucosa were found. Close monitoring of these patients must be carried out to observe the evolution of the process.

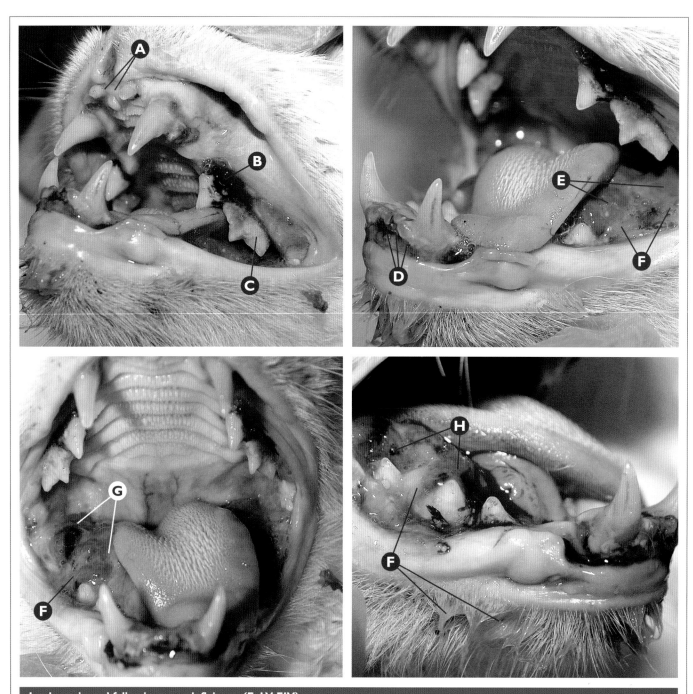

Leukaemia and feline immunodeficiency (FeLV, FIV)

Severe gingivostomatitis due to immunodeficiency (FIV) and calicivirus (FCV) in a 10-year-old patient. Viral analysis (PCR): FeLV -, FIV +, FCV +, FHV -.

A From right to left: Absence of LmaxI1 (202) and LmaxI1 (201).

B Gingival index 3 in LmaxP3 (207).

C Plaque index 4 on LmaxP4 (208).

D Gingival index 3 in LmandI1 (301), LmandI2 (302) and LmandI3 (303).

E Hyperplastic sublingual tissue in the lingual area of LmandP4 (308) and LmandM1 (309), which are both absent.

F Seropurulent fluid mixed with saliva.

G Hyperplastic tissue in the sublingual area and right caudal buccal mucosa.

H Image of the hyperplastic sublingual tissue, in the lingual area of RmandP4 (408) and RmandM1 (409).

Key diagnostic/treatment points

In this clinical case, feline immunodeficiency (FIV) and calicivirus (FCV) cause the syndrome, together with the highly patent and advanced periodontal disease. In these cases, the correct treatment of the periodontal disease (by means of adequate periodontal treatment and the extraction of the indicated teeth) and the control of the clinical signs of the viral infections are key to successfully treat the gingivostomatitis. Confirmation of the benign nature of the oral masses (after adequate histopathological diagnosis) is an indispensable step in this process.

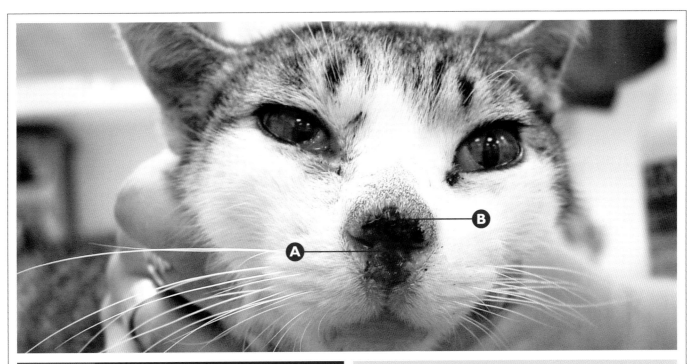

Neoplasms | **Squamous cell carcinoma**

Squamous cell carcinoma on the nose.

Ⓐ Ulceration and destruction of tissue.

Ⓑ Formation of scabs.

Key diagnostic/treatment points

Squamous cell carcinoma is a common malignant neoplasm in cats. It is frequently located on skin that has previously been damaged by the sun, which is why its incidence is greater in white-haired cats. It is most commonly located on the tip of the nose, pinnae, eyelids and lips. Treatment must be aggressive and early.

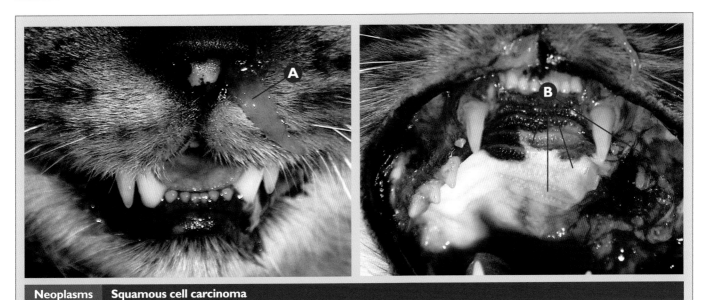

Neoplasms | **Squamous cell carcinoma**

Squamous cell carcinoma in the middle and distal third of the palate, affecting the area of the premolars and upper left molar (histopathologically confirmed).

Ⓐ Drainage of seropurulent fluid through the left nostril.

Ⓑ Neoplastic growth in the middle and distal third of the palate (squamous cell carcinoma), affecting the oral and nasal cavities.

Key diagnostic/treatment points

Squamous cell carcinoma is the most frequent malignant tumour in the oral cavity of cats; it is locally invasive with a great osteolytic regional metastatic capacity. Squamous cell carcinomas of the tonsils have a high regional and distant metastatic capacity. A histopathological diagnosis is indispensable. Treatment is radical surgery (with broad margins) with the possibility of radiotherapy depending on the location, with poor prognosis.

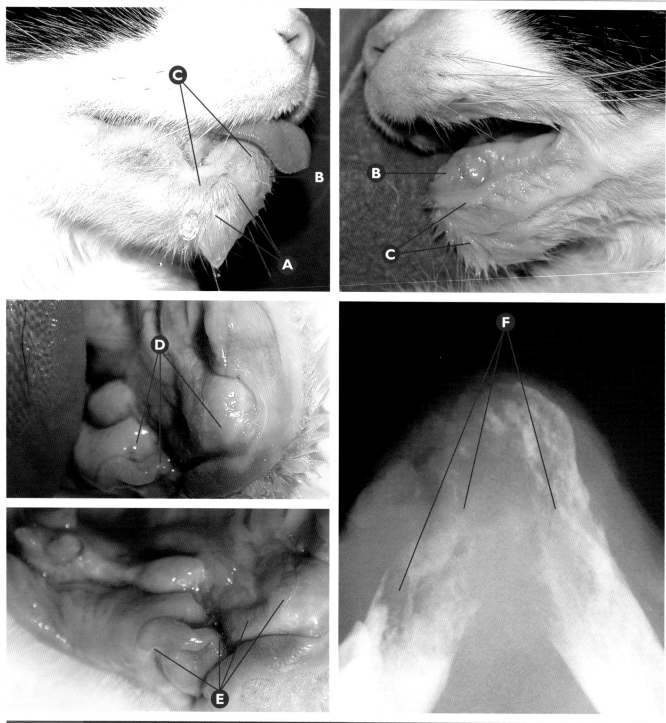

Neoplasms **Squamous cell carcinoma**

Squamous cell carcinoma in the area of the symphysis and lower canine teeth (histopathologically confirmed).

Ⓐ Inflammation/growth in the chin area.

Ⓑ Shortening of both mandibles in the rostral region.

Ⓒ Severe sialorrhea.

Ⓓ Absence of canine and lower incisor teeth.

Ⓔ Image of the absence of the canine and lower incisor teeth, with a lesion in the region of the absent RmandC (404).

Ⓕ Dental X-ray: radiological signs compatible with severe osteolysis in the area of the mandibular symphysis and lower canine teeth.

Key diagnostic/treatment points

Squamous cell carcinoma is the most frequent malignant tumour in the oral cavity of cats. In many cases, X-rays reveal a degree of invasion that greatly surpasses the macroscopic appearance of the process. The diagnosis must be made by means of a biopsy. The prognosis in these advanced cases is poor.

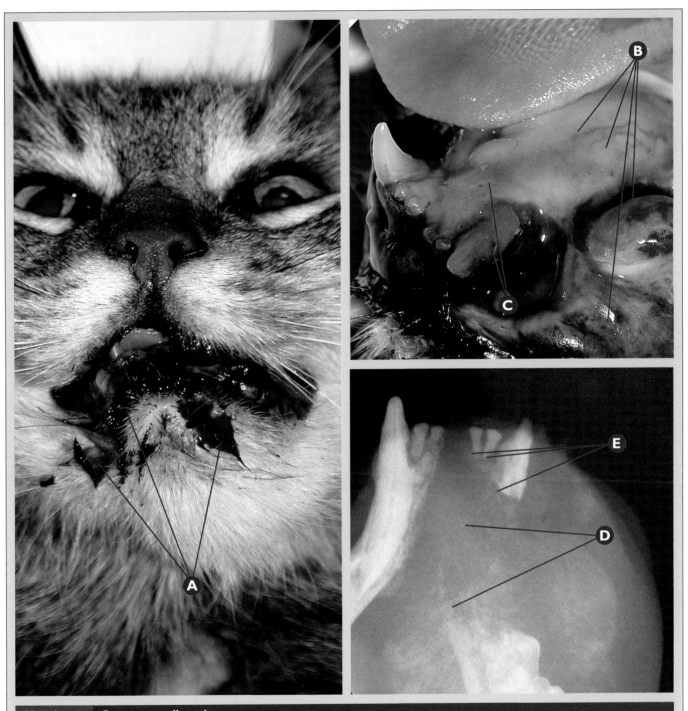

Neoplasms | Squamous cell carcinoma

Squamous cell carcinoma in the area of the symphysis and lower canine teeth (histopathologically confirmed).

Ⓐ Serosanguineous fluid mixed with saliva on the chin area.

Ⓑ Growth of a mass (squamous cell carcinoma) in the distolingual, distovestibular and distal areas of LmandC (304).

Ⓒ Suspicions of a root fracture of LmandC (304), with severe regional ulceration.

Ⓓ Dental X-ray: radiological signs compatible with severe osteolysis in the area of LmandC (304).

Ⓔ Dental X-ray: radiological signs compatible with severe dental destruction of LmandI2 (302), LmandI3 (303), and LmandC (304).

Key diagnostic/treatment points
Squamous cell carcinomas cause local bone destruction typical of malignant tumours. On many occasions, these neoplasms destroy dental tissue, sometimes aggressively. A histopathological diagnosis is indispensable, irrespective of the dental radiological findings, as these are only indicative for the diagnosis.

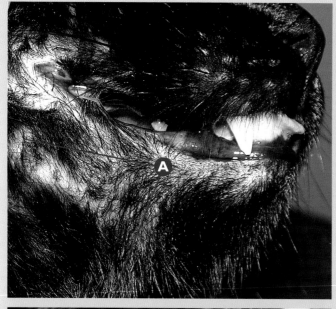

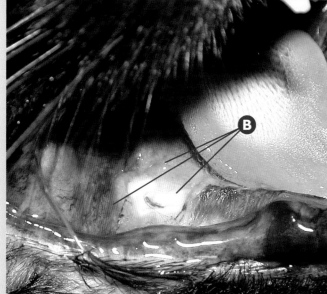

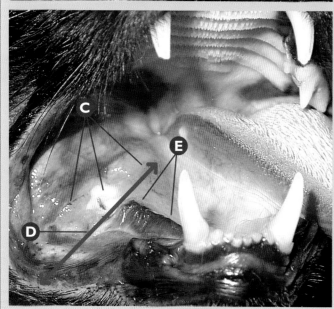

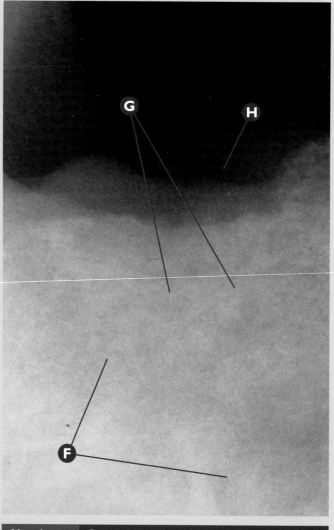

Neoplasms · **Squamous cell carcinoma**

Squamous cell carcinoma in the area of the absent RmandM1 (409) (histopathologically confirmed).

Ⓐ Severe thickening of the body of the mandible on the right side.

Ⓑ Severe ulcer with suspicions of bone exposure, surrounded by regional growth (squamous cell carcinoma).

Ⓒ Image of the squamous cell carcinoma in the area of the absent RmandM1 (409).

Ⓓ Severe mandibular thickening.

Ⓔ Absence of RmandP4 (408) and RmandP3 (407).

Ⓕ Dental X-ray: radiological signs compatible with severe diffuse osteolysis in the mandibular cortical bone, and severe osteoid thickening.

Ⓖ Dental X-ray: radiological signs compatible with moderate diffuse osteolysis.

Ⓗ Dental X-ray: radiological signs compatible with the absence of RmandM1 (409).

Key diagnostic/treatment points
Areas of compensatory thickening can also be detected in cases of squamous cell carcinomas due to the bone destruction that takes place (diffuse in this case). The dental macroscopic and radiological signs may be compatible with a focal osteomyelitis, which highlights the importance of always performing a histopathological analysis.

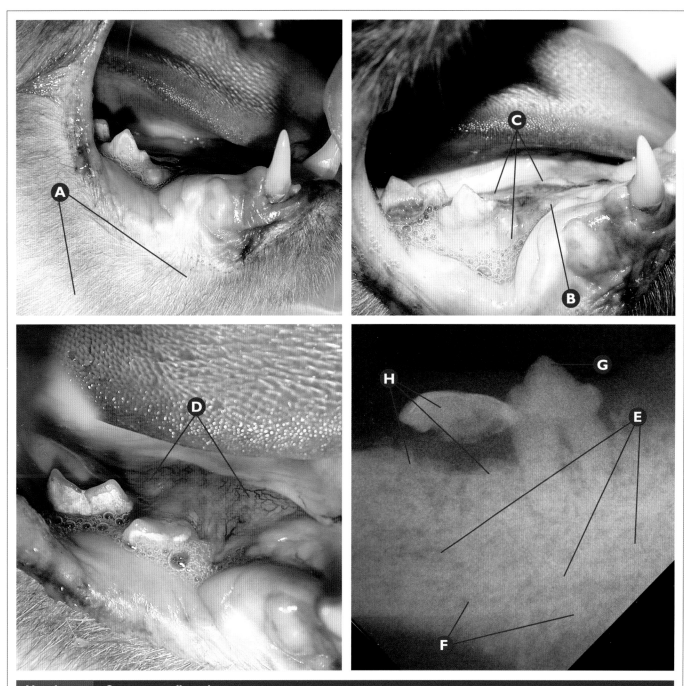

Neoplasms | Squamous cell carcinoma

Squamous cell carcinoma in the right mandibular body (histopathologically confirmed).

Ⓐ Severe thickening of the body of the mandible on the right side.

Ⓑ Suspicions of a coronal remnant of RmandP3 (407).

Ⓒ Mandibular thickening due to the growth of a vascularised mass in the lingual area of RmandP4 (408).

Ⓓ Close-up of the mandibular thickening, squamous cell carcinoma in the lingual area of RmandP4 (408).

Ⓔ Dental X-ray: radiological signs compatible with moderate diffuse osteolysis in the body of the right mandible.

Ⓕ Dental X-ray: radiological signs compatible with severe diffuse osteolysis in the mandibular cortical bone.

Ⓖ Dental X-ray: radiological signs compatible with RmandP4 (408).

Ⓗ Dental X-ray: radiological signs compatible with the crown (absence of roots) of RmandM1 (409).

Key diagnostic/treatment points
The macroscopic appearance and dental radiological signs of squamous cell carcinoma are highly variable. It causes bone destruction, which in this case is diffuse, and radiological areas compatible with compensatory areas can be observed. A histopathological study of the lesion is indispensable to make a correct diagnosis.

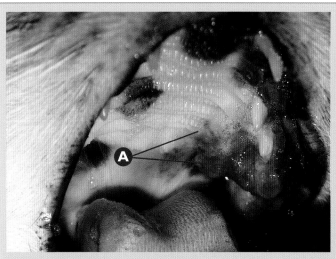

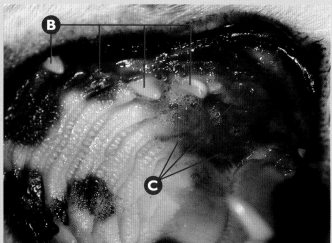

Neoplasms   Fibrosarcoma

Fibrosarcoma in gingiva and regional mucosa of LmaxP4 (208) (histopathologically confirmed).

Ⓐ Fibrosarcoma in gingiva and regional mucosa of LmaxP4 (208).

Ⓑ From right to left: LmaxP4 (208), LmaxP3 (207), LmaxP2 (206) and LmaxC (204).

Ⓒ Image of the fibrosarcoma in the gingiva and regional mucosa of LmaxP4 (208).

Key diagnostic/treatment points
Fibrosarcoma is the second most frequent tumour in the oral cavity of cats. It is a malignant tumour with little regional and distant metastatic capacity, in spite of being very invasive locally. Treatment is radical surgery with broad margins with a guarded prognosis. The radiographic margins of the neoplasm are determinant in the prognosis of the radical surgery.

Common errors
Assuming it is possible to diagnose oral neoplasms by means of a macroscopic oral examination. A histopathological analysis is essential to correctly diagnose oral neoplasms and rule out other non-neoplastic diseases.

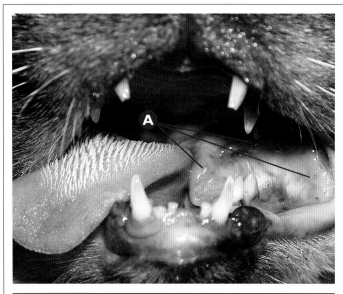

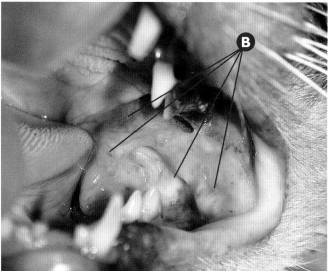

Neoplasms   Fibrosarcoma

Fibrosarcoma in the caudal buccal mucosa on the left side (histopathologically confirmed).

Ⓐ Fibrosarcoma in the caudal buccal mucosa on the left side, distal to LmandM1 (309).

Ⓑ Image of the fibrosarcoma in the caudal buccal mucosa on the left side.

Key diagnostic/treatment points
Fibrosarcoma is a very locally invasive malignant tumour as seen macroscopically in this clinical case. In spite of its low regional and distant metastatic capacity, in cases in which the location of the neoplasm makes radical surgical treatment difficult, such as in this clinical case, the prognosis is downgraded from guarded to poor.

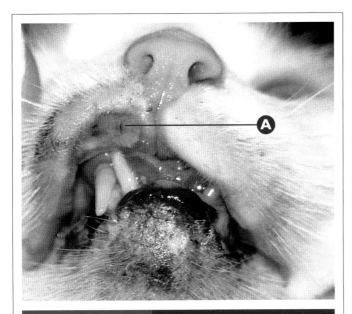

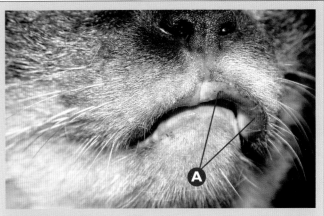

Metabolic, iatrogenic and other aetiologies	Eosinophilic granuloma

Feline eosinophilic granuloma on the upper right labial mucosa (histopathologically confirmed).

Ⓐ Image of the necrotic ulcer on the upper lip.

Key diagnostic/treatment points

Eosinophilic granulomas are mostly found in young cats, and can be uni- or bilateral. A differential diagnosis must be performed and include traumatic or neoplastic processes, thus making biopsy indispensable to diagnose this disease.

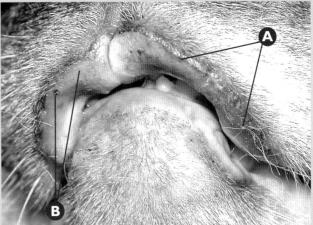

Metabolic, iatrogenic and other aetiologies	Eosinophilic granuloma

Feline eosinophilic granuloma on the left and right upper labial mucosa (histopathologically confirmed).

Ⓐ Feline eosinophilic granuloma on the left upper labial mucosa.

Ⓑ Feline eosinophilic granuloma on the right upper labial mucosa.

Ⓒ Follow-up, biopsy taking: feline eosinophilic granuloma on the upper left and right labial mucosa, eight days after the first visit.

Ⓓ Follow-up, biopsy taking: image of the granuloma at the same moment.

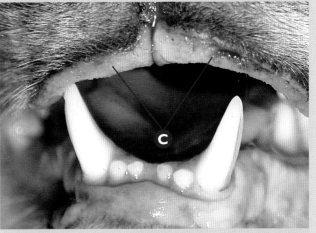

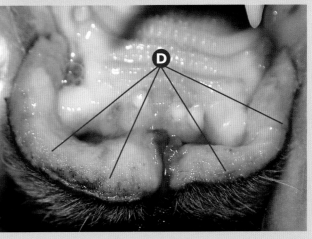

Key diagnostic/treatment points

Eosinophilic granulomas in cats must be confirmed by histopathological analysis to rule out other processes (neoplastic, traumatic, allergic...). Treatment is based on the administration of steroid anti-inflammatory drugs, and on the control of the secondary regional infection.

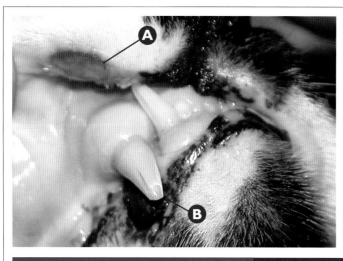

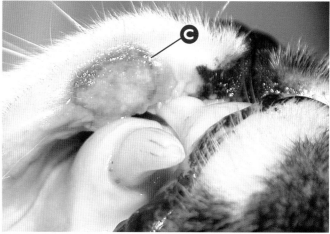

Metabolic, iatrogenic and other aetiologies | Eosinophilic granuloma

Feline eosinophilic granuloma on the right upper labial mucosa, rostral to RmaxC (104) (histopathologically confirmed).

Ⓐ Feline eosinophilic granuloma on the rostral labial mucosa in contact with RmaxC (104).

Ⓑ Suspicions of an uncomplicated crown fracture of RmaxC (104).

Ⓒ Image of the eosinophilic granuloma with the typical rounded and ulcerated appearance.

Key diagnostic/treatment points
Eosinophilic granulomas can occur in both cats and dogs, with only one or several lesions in the oral cavity. The typical location in cats is the upper lip. Although their appearance has been attributed to many factors (immune-mediated, infectious...), their true aetiology is unknown. A histopathological diagnosis is necessary to confirm the disease. Traditionally, treatment is based on the application of a corticosteroid therapy protocol, and good results are achieved.

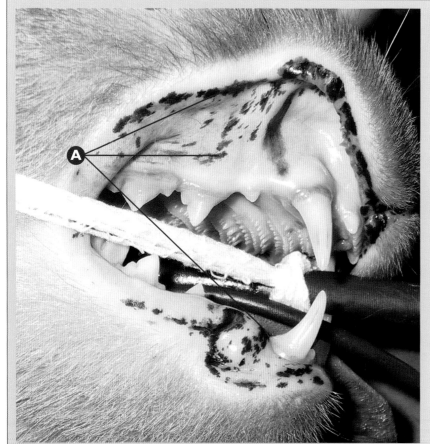

Metabolic, iatrogenic and other aetiologies
Lentigo

Feline lentigo

Ⓐ Image of the pigmentation in feline lentigo.

Key diagnostic/treatment points
In feline letigo, we can observe hyperpigmented spots in the vestibular and labial mucosa; this is typical in young tabby cats. This condition has no clinical or pathological significance.

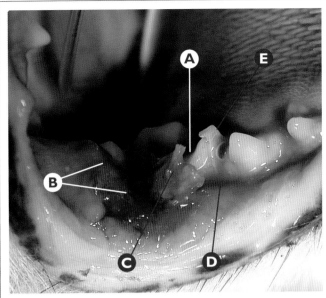

Severe lesion in the mucosa distal to RmandM1 (409) caused by a foreign body (grass awn).

Ⓐ RmandM1 (409).

Ⓑ Severe inflammation in the area distal to RmandM1 (409).

Ⓒ Suspicions of a foreign body.

Ⓓ Moderate inflammation of the mesiovestibular mucosa of RmandM1 (409).

Ⓔ Suspicions of a second foreign body.

Ⓕ Close-up of the severe inflammation in the area distal to RmandM1 (409).

Ⓖ Close-up of the grass awn after being removed from the oral cavity.

Ⓗ Image of a bone splinter after its removal from the mesial area of RmandM1 (409).

Key diagnostic/treatment points

Small-sized foreign bodies may become embedded in the soft tissues or interdental spaces, and go unnoticed. With time, they may cause mild to moderate signs compatible with oral pain. If their elimination is not adequate or is delayed, the regional soft tissues will inflame, which will favour the progression of the periodontal disease and cause signs of oral pain. The prognosis of this condition is good to guarded. Treatment is based on the elimination of the cause (foreign body removal), as well as on adequate antibiotic and anti-inflammatory treatment.

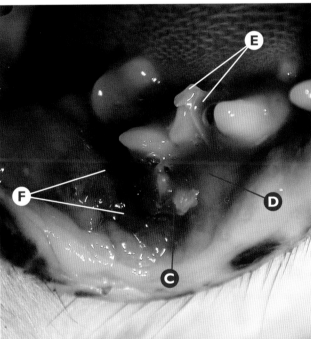

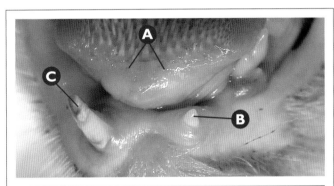

Severe lesion on the tongue from an electric cord burn, moderate loss of lingual tissue (see the "Electric cord burns" case).

Ⓐ Lingual lesion with scar tissue on the tip of the tongue, and loss of tissue from the electric cord burn.

Ⓑ Suspicions of the cusp of LmandC (304).

Ⓒ Signs of a burn on the cusp of RmandC (404).

Key diagnostic/treatment points

Electric cord burns may cause severe damage to the lingual tissue, including loss of tissue or changes to the shape of the tongue. These lesions do not normally change the tongue's function, except in those cases where the loss of lingual tissue is very severe.

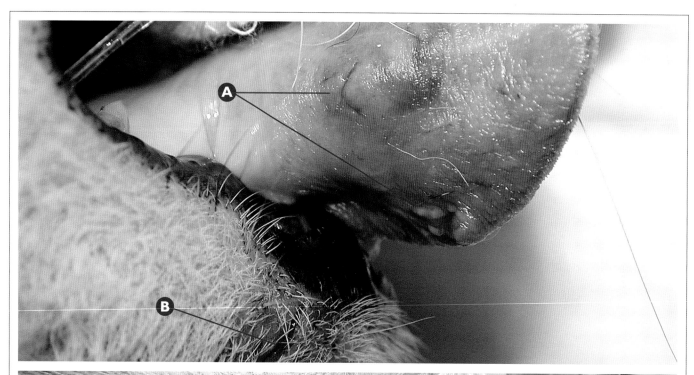

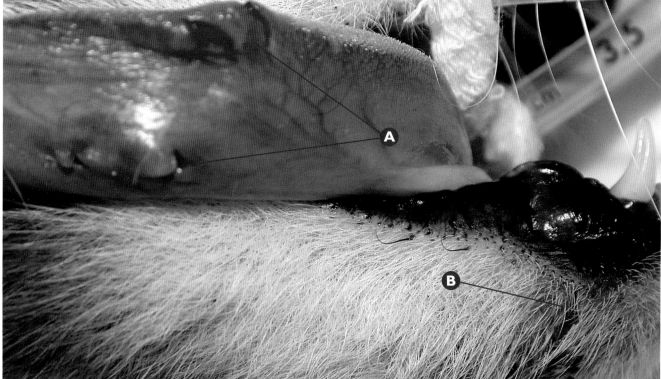

Traumatic aetiology | **Soft-tissue lesions** | **Tongue lesions**

Moderate lesion on the ventral surface of the tongue from self-biting when receiving external trauma to the oral cavity.

Ⓐ Injury on the ventral surface of the tongue from self-biting.

Ⓑ Injury to the skin of the lower lip in the area of RmandC (404) due to external trauma.

Key diagnostic/treatment points

Occasionally, in patients that have suffered external trauma (run over by a vehicle, fallen from great heights...), the trauma may have caused mild to severe injuries to both hard and soft tissues. Tongue injuries caused by the animal biting itself when suffering external trauma are one of these types of lesions in soft tissues. Most of these lesions have a good prognosis.

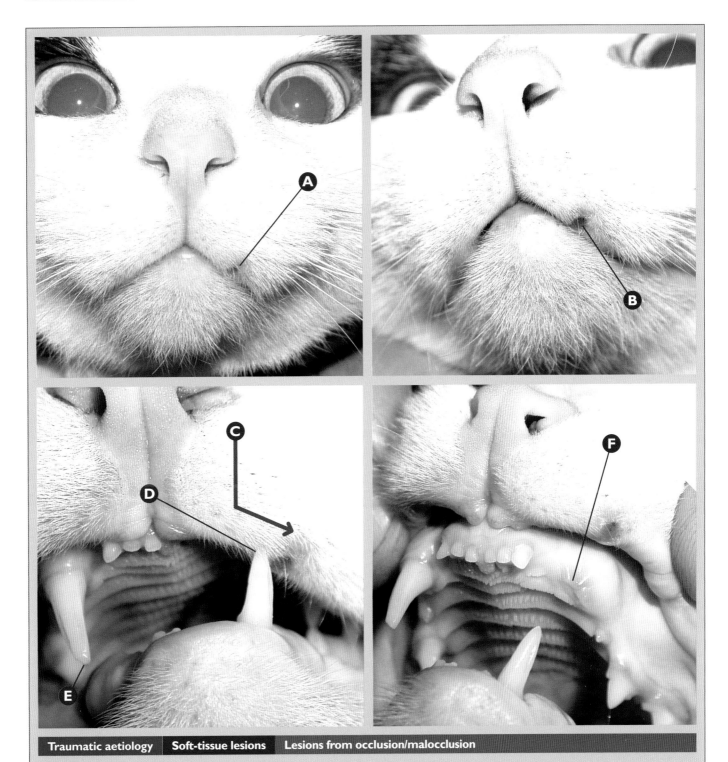

Traumatic aetiology | **Soft-tissue lesions** | **Lesions from occlusion/malocclusion**

Ulcerated lesion on the skin and labial mucosa in the area rostral to the absent LmaxC (204), due to impingement of its lower counterpart.

Ⓐ Ulcerated lesion on the skin and labial mucosa in the area rostral to LmaxC (204).

Ⓑ Image of the ulcerated lesion on the skin and labial mucosa in the area rostral to LmaxC (204).

Ⓒ Distal displacement of the upper lip on the left side.

Ⓓ Cusp of LmandC (304) occluding into the upper lip.

Ⓔ Suspicions of an uncomplicated crown fracture of RmaxC (104).

Ⓕ Absence of LmaxC (204), which facilitates the distal and palatal displacement of the upper lip on the left side.

Key diagnostic/treatment points

Lesions in soft tissues due to inadequate occlusion are relatively frequent in cats, especially those caused by missing teeth, which facilitate lesions due to malocclusion. Adequate treatment for this clinical case would be crown reduction of LmandC (304) by means of a partial coronal pulpectomy. Occlusal and intraoral lateral X-rays of the maxilla are highly recommended to evaluate the existence or absence of a retained root of LmaxC (204).

49

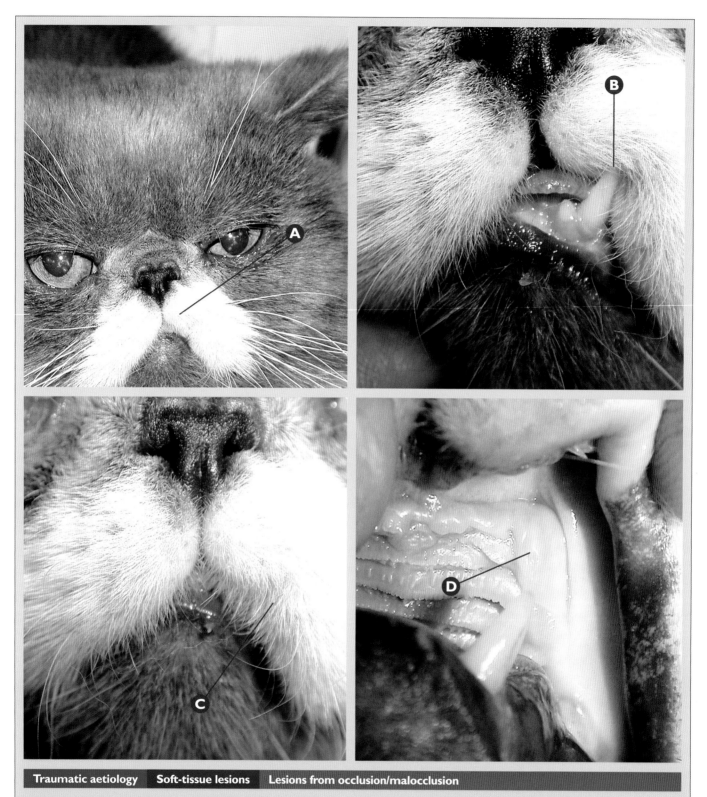

Traumatic aetiology | **Soft-tissue lesions** | **Lesions from occlusion/malocclusion**

Mild lesion on the skin and labial mucosa in the area rostral to absent LmaxC (204), due to impingement of LmandC (304) over this area.

Ⓐ Appearance of the animal at rest. LmandC (304) slightly occludes into the upper lip.

Ⓑ Close-up of LmandC (304) occluding into the upper lip.

Ⓒ Close-up of the mild lesion on the skin of the upper lip, after resolving the malocclusion of LmandC (304) by manually moving the upper lip in a rostral direction.

Ⓓ Absence of LmaxC (204).

Key diagnostic/treatment points
The absence of the upper canine teeth (due to agenesis, previous extraction or any other cause), occasionally causes the upper lip to rest in a distal direction, which facilitates the occlusion of the lower canine tooth into the lip. Appropriate treatment should be provided to avoid constant trauma to the lip area.

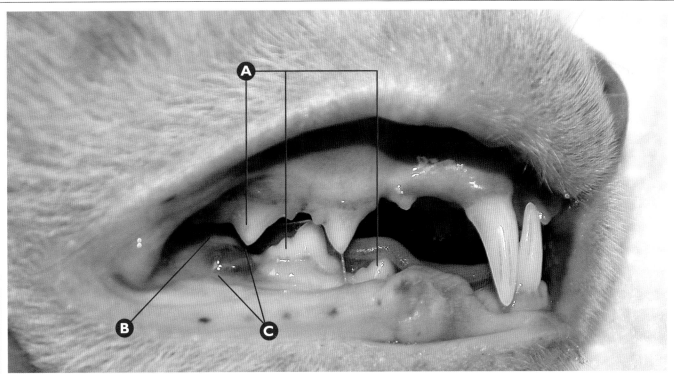

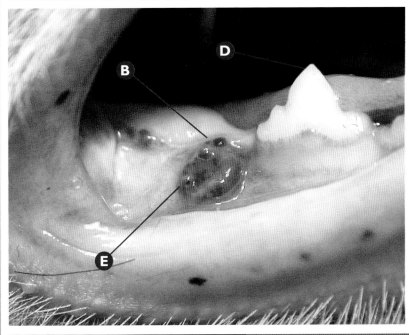

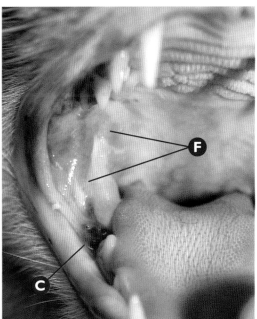

Traumatic aetiology **Soft-tissue lesions** **Lesions from occlusion/malocclusion**

Severe lesion in the mucosa of the area of the absent RmandM1 (409), due to occlusion of RmaxP4 (108) into this region.

A From right to left: RmandP1 (407), RmandP4 (408) and RmaxP4 (108).

B Absence of RmandM1(409).

C Severe lesion in the mucosa of the area of the absent RmandM1 (409), due to occlusion of RmaxP4 (108).

D RmandP4 (408).

E Close-up of the ulcer in the mucosa of the area of RmandM1 (409).

F Absence of regional lesions, especially in the caudal buccal mucosa on the right side.

Key diagnostic/treatment points

Occasionally, when RmandM1 (409) is missing (after extraction, for example), RmaxP4 (108) may occlude into the regional mandibular mucosa and cause lesions, especially ulcers or granulation tissue from the trauma. The extraction of RmaxP4 (108) is one of the options to be considered to avoid this constant trauma. An incisional biopsy of the area is highly recommended to rule out any neoplastic processes and confirm the traumatic origin of the lesion.

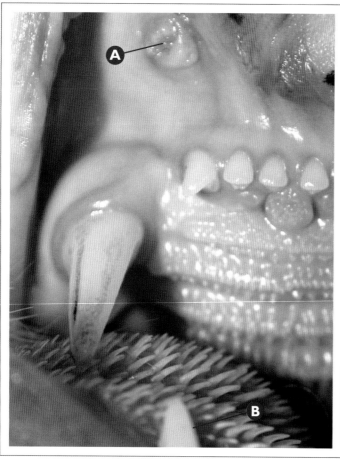

Traumatic aetiology

Soft-tissue lesions
Lesions from occlusion/malocclusion

Ulcerated lesion in the mucosa of the upper lip, in the area apical to RmaxI3 (103), due to the occlusion of RmandC (404) into this area.

Ⓐ Ulcerated lesion in the mucosa of the area apical to RmaxI3 (103).

Ⓑ Cusp of RmandC (404) that occludes into the mucosa of the upper lip when closing the oral cavity.

Key diagnostic/treatment points
When we detect different types of malocclusions, we may also detect lesions in the soft tissues caused by the changes to the normal physiological occlusion. Treatment should be based on the elimination of the traumatic cause and control of any local infection.

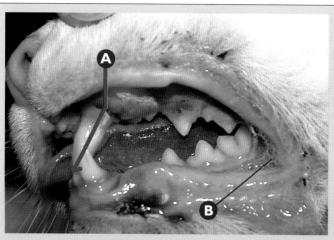

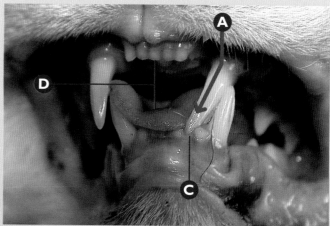

Traumatic aetiology | **Soft-tissue lesions** | **Lesions from occlusion/malocclusion**

Moderate lesion caused by the occlusion of LmaxC (204) into the gingiva. The tooth is displaced due to suspected severe periodontal disease and causes the displacement of the lower incisor teeth.

Ⓐ Mesiopalatal displacement of LmaxC (204) due to suspected severe periodontal disease.

Ⓑ Sialorrhea.

Ⓒ Moderate lesion between LmandI2 (302) and LmandI3 (303) with displacement of both teeth due to malocclusion of the cusp of the displaced LmaxC (204).

Ⓓ Inability to close the oral cavity.

Key diagnostic/treatment points
In this clinical case, the soft-tissue lesion is caused by malocclusion of a displaced upper canine tooth, which is likely a consequence of severe periodontal disease (tooth resorption must be ruled out for this tooth). This causes a soft-tissue lesion and inability to close the oral cavity with the resulting pain. Occlusal and intraoral lateral X-rays of the maxilla must be taken to determine the exact cause of the displacement of LmaxC (204); extraction of the tooth is the most common non-conservative treatment.

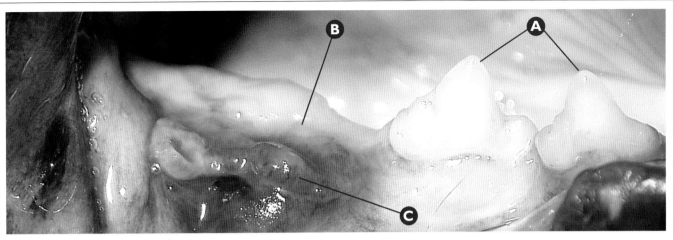

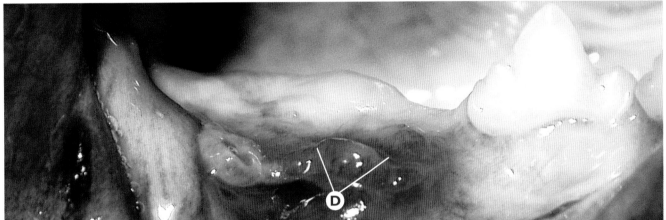

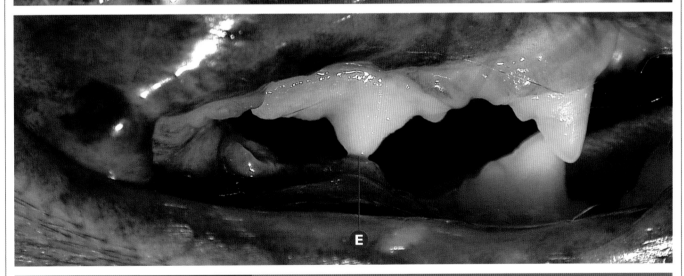

Traumatic aetiology | **Soft-tissue lesions** | **Lesions from occlusion/malocclusion**

Severe lesion in the mucosa of the area of the absent RmandM1 (409), due to occlusion of RmaxP4 (108) into this region.

Ⓐ From right to left: RmandP3 (407) and RmandP4 (408).

Ⓑ Absence of RmandM1(409).

Ⓒ Severe ulcer in the mucosa of the vestibular area of the absent RmandM1 (409).

Ⓓ Image of the severe ulcer in the mucosa of the vestibular area of the absent RmandM1 (409), with the mark caused by the occlusion of RmaxP4 (108).

Ⓔ Image of the occlusion of RmaxP4 (108) into the vestibular mucosa of the absent RmandM1 (409).

Key diagnostic/treatment points
This clinical case is yet another example of how the absence of a first lower molar may cause lesions due to the occlusion of the fourth upper premolar. Occasionally, the extraction of the latter is the only effective treatment option to resolve these lesions (elimination of the traumatic cause).

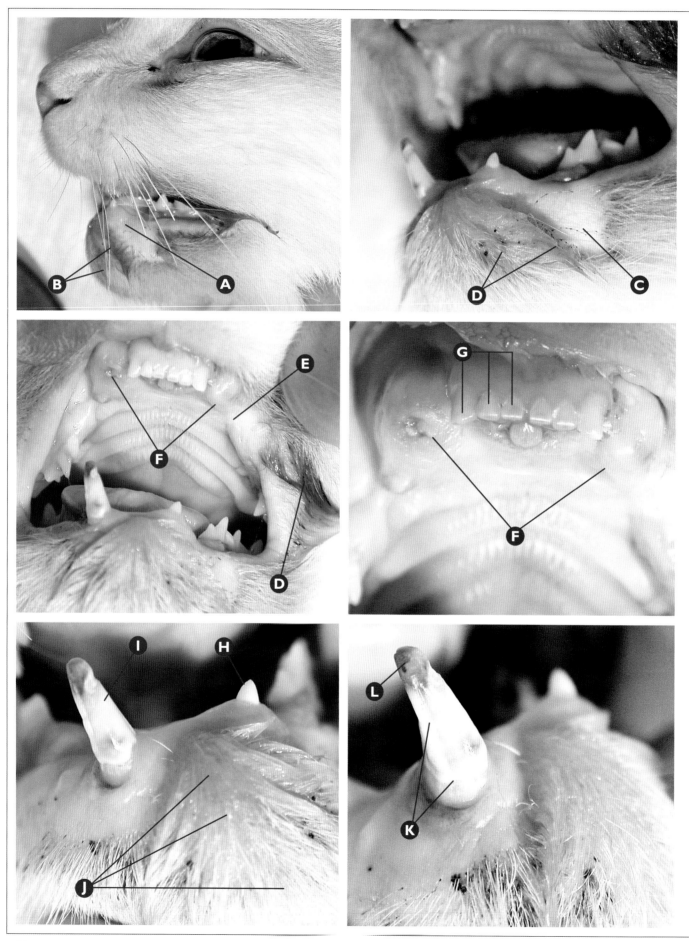

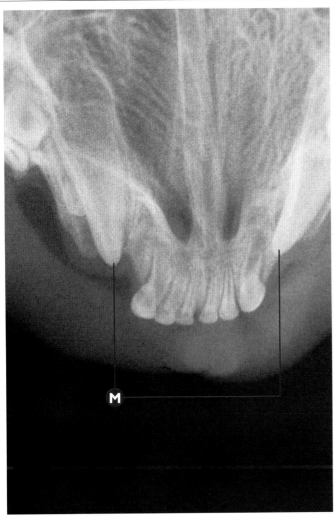

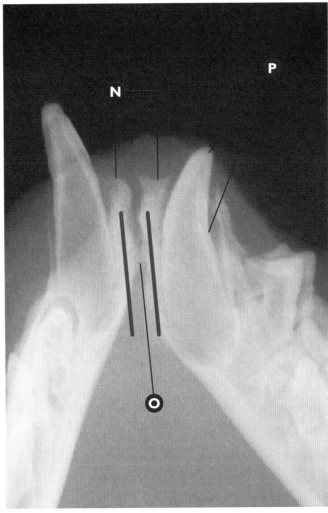

Traumatic aetiology | **Soft-tissue lesions** | **Electric cord burn**

Lesions from electric cord burns, causing injuries to soft tissues and changes in the genesis and eruption of permanent teeth.

Ⓐ Scarred lesion in the mucosa and skin of the lower lip in the region of LmandC (304).

Ⓑ Moderate inflammation in the chin area of the left mandible.

Ⓒ Close-up of the scarred lesion in the mucosa and skin of the lower lip in the region of LmandC (304).

Ⓓ Increase in the density of the saliva; its seropurulent appearance leads us to suspect the existence of an infection.

Ⓔ Severe scarred lesion in the mucosa and skin of the lower lip in the region of LmaxC (204).

Ⓕ Absence of the upper permanent and deciduous canine teeth.

Ⓖ From right to left: RmaxI1 (101), RmaxI2 (102), RmaxI3 (103).

Ⓗ Suspicions of the cusp of LmandC (304).

Ⓘ RmandC (404).

Ⓙ Moderate-severe inflammation in the chin area.

Ⓚ Suspected odontodysplasia of RmandC (404) from a regional electric burn.

Ⓛ Signs of a burn on the cusp of RmandC (404).

Ⓜ Dental X-ray: (from right to left) radiological signs compatible with LmaxC (204) and RmaxC (104), without erupting.

Ⓝ Dental X-ray: radiological signs compatible with the absence of the lower incisor teeth.

Ⓞ Dental X-ray: radiological signs compatible with severe changes to the bone in the mandibular symphysis.

Ⓟ Dental X-ray: radiological signs compatible with delayed dental eruption and severe changes to the periodontal ligament in LmandC (304).

Key diagnostic/treatment points

Electric cord burns, which normally occur after suffering a shock from chewing on a cord, are typical in young animals. This shock may cause severe lesions in regional soft and hard tissues, as well as changes in the development of the dental germ, which may affect tooth structure and eruption. Dental radiological studies in the short and mid-term are indispensable to control the evolution and consequences of the lesions. Treatment in these animals must focus on reestablishing the functionality of the oral cavity as well as preventing and treating any soft-tissue, bone and dental lesions.

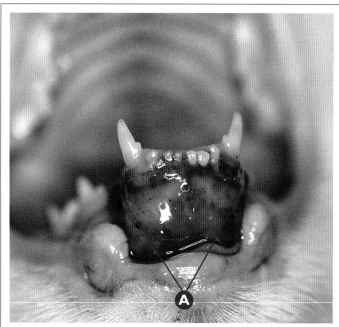

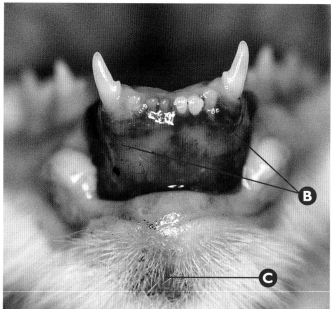

Traumatic aetiology | **Soft-tissue lesions** | **External trauma**

Moderate-severe avulsion of the lower lip in the chin region.

Ⓐ Avulsion of the lower lip in the chin region, bilateral.

Ⓑ Image of the avulsion of the lower lip in the chin region, with exposure of bone tissue.

Ⓒ Image of suspected traumatic injury.

Key diagnostic/treatment points

In those cases where the lesion is limited to soft tissues (after dental radiological study and confirmation) in specific locations such as in this clinical case, treatment is based on putting the soft tissues back into place, with a prognosis that ranges from guarded to very good.

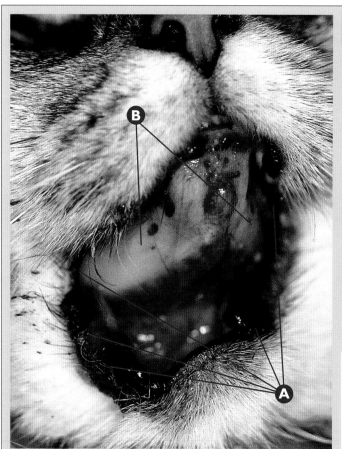

Traumatic aetiology | **Soft-tissue lesions** **External trauma**

Extreme avulsion of the lower lip of unknown traumatic origin.

Ⓐ Extreme avulsion of the lower lip.

Ⓑ Area of bone exposure of both sides of the mandible.

Key diagnostic/treatment points

In those cases in which only the soft tissues are affected, even extensively, and as long as the vascularisation is intact, the prognosis of recovery of the soft tissues is guarded to good. Adequate antibiotic, anti-inflammatory and analgesic therapy must be initiated before repair and continue during the postoperative period.

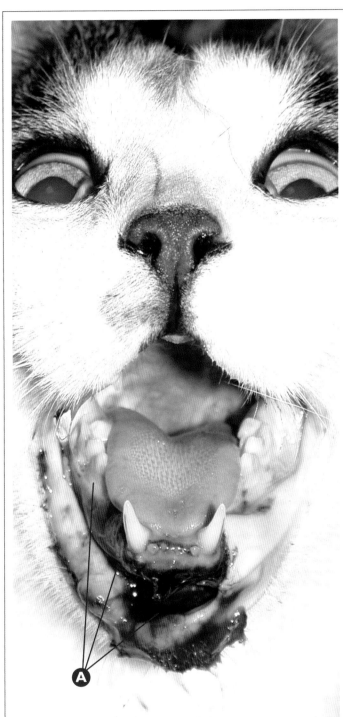

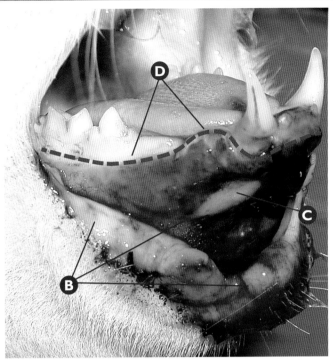

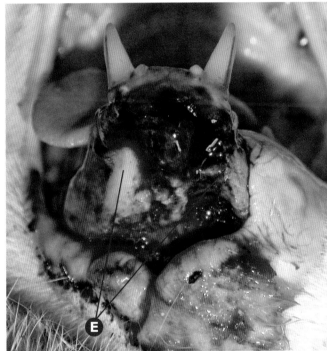

Traumatic aetiology | **Soft-tissue lesions** | **External trauma**

Severe lesion in the lower lip as a result of being run over by a vehicle.

Ⓐ Avulsion of the lower lip on the right side and symphyseal area.

Ⓑ Close-up of the avulsion of the lower lip on the right side, with exposure of bone tissue.

Ⓒ Right mandible.

Ⓓ Area of laceration of the mucosa caused by the trauma.

Ⓔ Close-up of the areas of bone exposure in the rostral region of both mandibles.

Key diagnostic/treatment points

In cases of severe trauma to the oral cavity such as that observed in this clinical case, it is important to assess the damage to hard and soft tissues. Conventional and dental radiography and, above all, computed tomography (CT) are the most appropriate diagnostic methods for a first assessment of the damage to the regional bone tissues. Treatment involves putting the hard and soft tissues back into place with different fixation systems, as well as adequate antibiotic, anti-inflammatory and analgesic therapy. The prognosis in these cases is highly variable; it is guarded on most occasions.

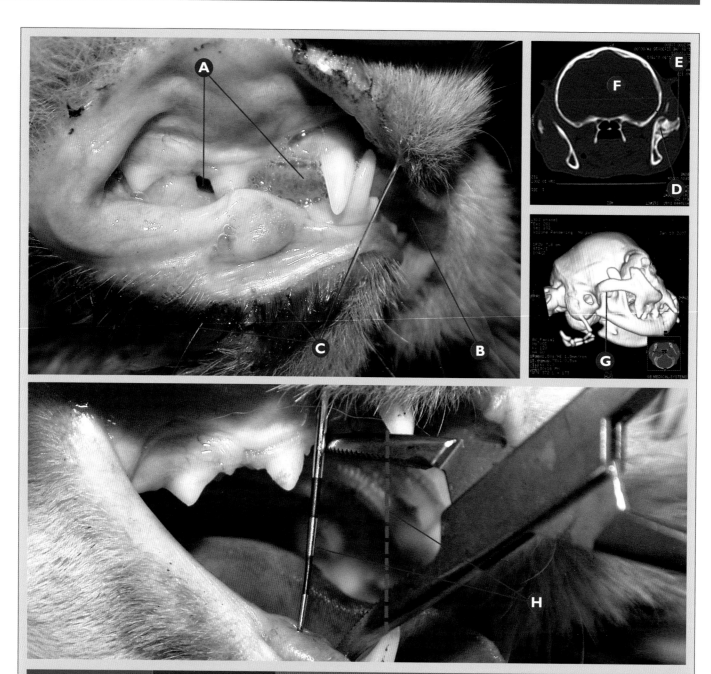

Traumatic aetiology | **Hard-tissue lesions** | **Fractures - trauma to the temporomandibular joint area - miscellaneous**

Inability to open the oral cavity in an 8-month-old patient, due to ankylosis of the right temporomandibular joint and fusion of the osteoid tissue to the zygomatic arch; previous trauma.

Ⓐ Complete closure of the oral cavity and inability to open it while under sedation.

Ⓑ Rostral portion of the tongue trapped in the incisor area.

Ⓒ Accumulation of saliva due to sialorrhea.

Ⓓ CT scan*: radiological signs compatible with ankylosis of the right temporo-mandibular joint and fusion of the osteoid tissue to the right zygomatic arch.

Ⓔ CT scan*: right zygomatic arch.

Ⓕ CT scan*: radiological signs compatible with an area of fusion with the right zygomatic arch.

Ⓖ 3D-CT scan*: image compatible with ankylosis of the right temporomandibular joint.

Ⓗ Immediate postoperative period: opening of the oral cavity greater than 12 mm (measured with a periodontal probe), immediately after the surgical resolution of the pathology.

* Acknowledgements to the Hospital Veterinari Marina Baixa Alicante (Spain), for providing these CT scan and 3D-CT scan images.

Key diagnostic/treatment points

In those clinical cases with previous trauma (or unknown history) and inability to open the oral cavity, complementary diagnostic tests must be performed to reach an adequate diagnosis. Conventional and dental X-rays provide us with very limited diagnostic information on many occasions. CT scans and 3D reconstructions offer diagnostic information that is indispensable in these cases.

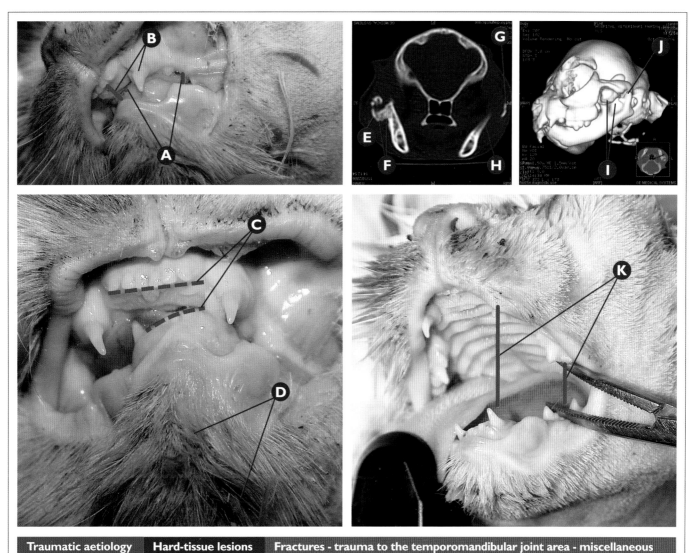

Traumatic aetiology | **Hard-tissue lesions** | **Fractures - trauma to the temporomandibular joint area - miscellaneous**

Inability to open the oral cavity in a 4-month-old patient caused by the fusion of the masseteric fossa of the left mandible to the zygomatic arch resulting from the formation of osteoid tissue; history of trauma when the animal was 1.5 months old.

🅐 Complete closure of the oral cavity with inability to open it under sedation.

🅑 Suspected mandibular distocclusion, with visible malocclusion of the deciduous LmandC (704) in the palatal area of the deciduous LmaxC (604).

🅒 Suspicions of acquired maxillomandibular asymmetry in a rostrocaudal direction with deviation of the midline.

🅓 Moderate accumulation of saliva due to sialorrhea.

🅔 CT scan*: left zygomatic arch.

🅕 CT scan*: radiological signs compatible with fusion of the masseteric fossa of the left mandible to the zygomatic arch due to the formation of osteoid tissue.

🅖 CT scan*: right zygomatic arch.

🅗 CT scan*: radiological signs compatible with the masseteric fossa of the right mandible.

🅘 3D-CT scan*: image compatible with osteoid tissue that fuses the masseteric fossa of the left mandible to the zygomatic arch.

🅙 3D-CT scan*: image compatible with mild changes to the normal morphology of the temporomandibular joint.

🅚 Immediate postoperative period: opening of the oral cavity immediately after the surgical resolution of the pathology.

* Acknowledgements to the Hospital Veterinari Marina Baixa Alicante (Spain), for providing these CT scan and 3D-CT scan images.

Key diagnostic/treatment points
Special care should be taken to correctly diagnose those patients that present with an inability to open the oral cavity (especially those with a history of trauma). Due to the limited (and often confusing) information that conventional X-rays provide in these clinical cases, CT and its 3D reconstructions become indispensable for the correct diagnosis of these processes. In this clinical case, the inability to open the oral cavity is caused by the newly formed osteoid tissue and not by any changes to the temporomandibular joints (confirmed during treatment by opening the oral cavity after eliminating the osteoid tissue from the pathological fusion).

Common errors
Assuming that the inability to open the oral cavity in feline patients with a history of trauma is based on the changes caused to the temporomandibular joint or any of its structures. The use of a CT scan for diagnosis in these cases is essential.

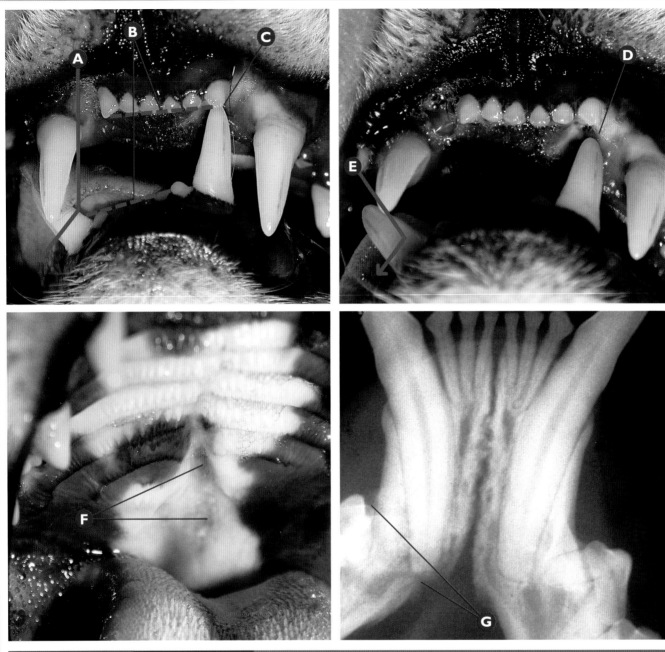

Traumatic aetiology | **Hard-tissue lesions** | **Mandibular fractures**

Suspected bilateral non-recent mandibular fracture in the distal area of RmandC (404); malocclusion due to inadequate resolution of the mandibular fracture.

A Malocclusion, with displacement of the mandible towards the right side; rostral view.

B Suspicions of maxillomandibular asymmetry in a dorsoventral direction.

C Impingement of the cusp of LmandC (304) into the distal region of Lmaxl3 (203).

D Image of the occlusion of the cusp of LmandC (304) into the distal region of Lmaxl3 (203).

E Distal displacement of RmandC (404) that causes it to occlude distally from RmaxC (104), due to a suspected mandibular fracture.

F Mild ulcer from recent closure of a wound in the mucosa of the soft and hard palates.

G Dental X-ray: radiological signs compatible with mandibular fracture distal to RmandC (404).

Key diagnostic/treatment points

When a mandibular fracture is detected in a cat, its surgical resolution is of utmost importance not only for the obvious reasons, but because of the high probability of moderate to severe malocclusion that frequently impedes adequate closure of the oral cavity. In this clinical case, surgical resolution of the mandibular fracture was not carried out when the trauma was recent, thus causing a visible malocclusion.

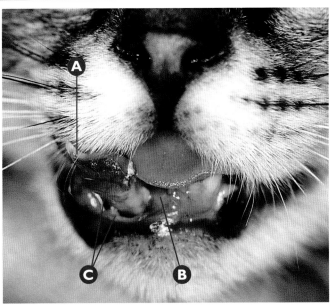

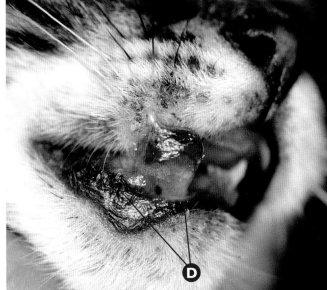

Traumatic aetiology   **Hard-tissue lesions**   **Mandibular fractures**

Symphyseal separation with avulsion of the lower lip in a 4-month-old patient.

Ⓐ Deciduous RmandC (804).

Ⓑ Symphyseal separation.

Ⓒ Severe right lip avulsion, with bone exposure.

Ⓓ Image of the right lip avulsion.

Key diagnostic/treatment points

In the case of polytraumatised animals with bone lesions in the oral cavity, conventional and dental X-rays as well as a CT scan should be performed to assess all damage and select the most adequate surgical resolution of the fractures.

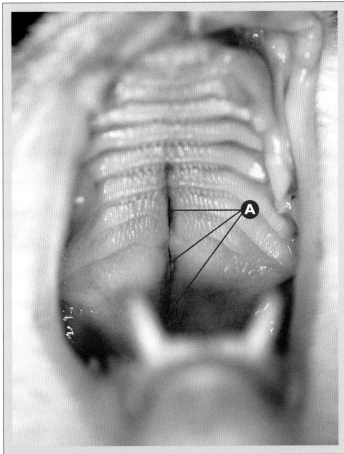

Traumatic aetiology   **Hard-tissue lesions**   **Maxillary fractures**

Suspected maxillary fracture caused from a fall from great heights.

Ⓐ Linear wound in the soft and hard palates.

Key diagnostic/treatment points

When a maxillary fracture is suspected, dental X-rays should be the first diagnostic step to be taken to assess the scope of the bone tissue lesion. If there is no significant displacement of the bone tissues of the palate in the fracture, treatment will be focused on preventing and treating palatal fissures and oronasal fistulae. The lesion shown in this clinical case is frequently detected in the cases of patients that have fallen from great heights.

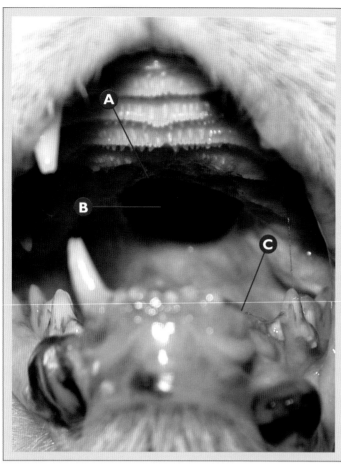

Traumatic aetiology | Hard-tissue lesions / Maxillary fractures

Consequence of a previous maxillary fracture that has become chronic, causing an acquired oronasal fistula in the soft and hard palates.

Ⓐ Severe oronasal fistula in the soft and hard palates.

Ⓑ Nasal cavity.

Ⓒ Absence of LmandC (304).

Key diagnostic/treatment points
When maxillary fractures are not treated, oronasal fistulae frequently appear. Acquired oronasal fistulae must be confirmed in the definitive oral examination with the animal under anaesthesia, including a dental radiological study (with a CT scan for some cases) to determine the true extent of the fistula. The signs detected in these cases are those typically associated with the entry of food into the nasal cavity (rhinitis, sneezing, difficulty eating). Surgical resolution of the condition is indicated with a guarded prognosis.

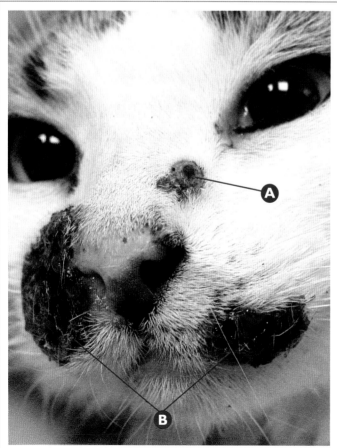

Bacterial, viral, fungal and parasitic origin | Cryptococcosis

Cryptococcosis.

Ⓐ Papulonodular lesion on the tip of the nose.

Ⓑ Ulcerative and scabby nodular lesions on the left upper lip and on the right side in the area adjacent to the nose.

Key diagnostic/treatment points
Facial lesions caused by *Cryptococcus neoformans*. The dermatological pattern observed in this animal corresponds with a nodular pattern with a tendency to ulcerate.

When dealing with nodular lesions, the most probable differential diagnoses would be as follows: neoplasm (multiple mastocytoma, sebaceous or apocrine gland carcinoma, squamous cell carcinoma...), infectious granuloma of fungal origin (sporotrichosis, phaeohyphomycosis, dermatophytic pseudomycetoma, cryptococcosis) or bacterial (botryomycosis, actinomycotic mycetoma, nocardiosis, mycobacteria) or multiple abscesses.

The first and primary test that should be performed in these cases is a cytological analysis. A cytological examination will determine whether the process is neoplastic, inflammatory or infectious. In this case, the cytological examination showed the presence of numerous encapsulated spheric formations compatible with *Cryptococcus* spp.

Common errors
Not performing complementary examinations. Feline cryptococcosis is usually associated with immunocompromised statuses, related or not to other diseases. In cats it is important to rule out infections by the feline immunodeficiency virus infection, feline leukaemia virus, and *Toxoplasma gondii*.

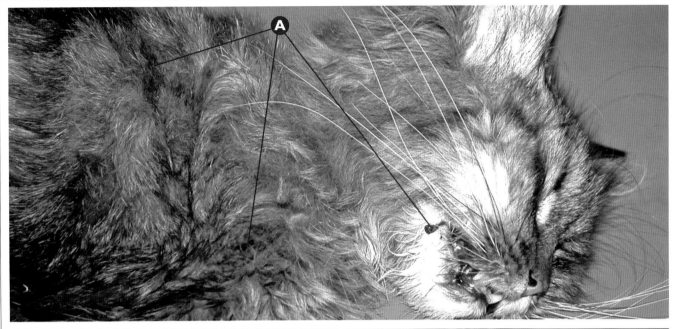

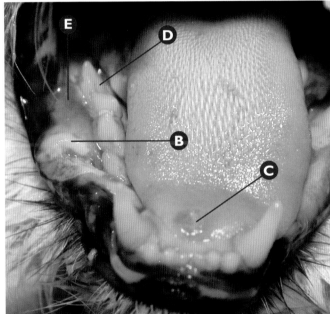

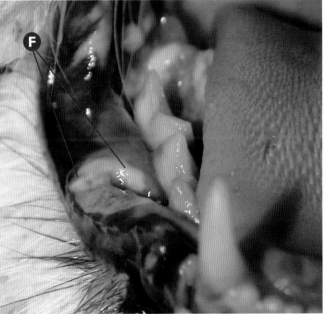

Bacterial, viral, fungal and parasitic origin | **Candidiasis**

Candidiasis (*Candida* spp.) in the oral mucosa of a cat with feline immunodeficiency (FIV), treated with long-term antibiotic and corticosteroid therapy (confirmed by means of microscopic visualisation of hyphae).

Ⓐ Signs of systemic immunodepression (quality of fur, weight loss) in a patient with FIV.

Ⓑ White coloured ulcerated lesion typical of the lesions caused by candidiasis.

Ⓒ Suspected lesion by candidiasis on the dorsal surface of the tongue.

Ⓓ RmandM1 (409).

Ⓔ Suspected stomatitis in the vestibular mucosa of RmandM1 (409).

Ⓕ Image of the lesion by candidiasis in the vestibular mucosa.

Key diagnostic/treatment points

Oral candidiasis is a fungal pathology caused in most cases by *Candida albicans*. It occurs in both dogs and cats in locations such as the lips and tongue, although it is uncommon. The most common cause of this disease is the patient having an immunocompromised system, as well as treatments with continued antibiotic and/or corticosteroid therapy. For this reason, it is detected relatively frequently in patients on these kinds of treatment to control feline gingivostomatitis. Typical signs include "white plaques" and a tendency to bleed in the surrounding ulcerated area. Diagnosis is based on the visualisation of hyphae after staining and/or a culture in specific media. The importance of the disease lies in its capacity to infect humans (zoonosis). Treatment is based on systemic antifungal therapy.

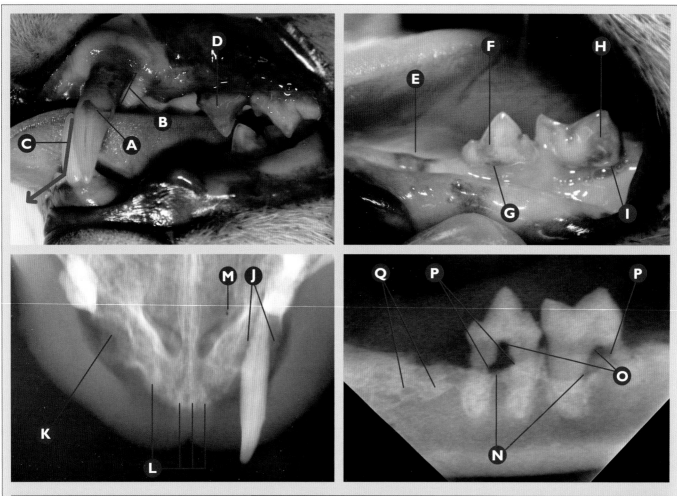

Bacterial, viral, fungal and parasitic origin | Periodontal disease

Stage 4 periodontal disease in LmaxC (204), LmandP4 (308) and LmandM1 (309).

Ⓐ Calculus index 1 on LmaxC (204).

Ⓑ Extrusion of LmaxC (204), due to periodontal disease.

Ⓒ Mesiovestibular displacement of LmaxC (204), due to periodontal disease.

Ⓓ Calculus index 4 on LmaxP3 (207).

Ⓔ Absence of LmandP3 (307).

Ⓕ Calculus index 2 on LmandP4 (308).

Ⓖ Gingival index 1 in LmandP4 (308).

Ⓗ Calculus index 3 on LmandM1 (309).

Ⓘ Gingival index 2 in the area of LmandM1 (309).

Ⓙ Dental X-ray: radiological signs compatible with stage 4 periodontal disease in LmaxC (204).

Ⓚ Dental X-ray: radiological signs compatible with absence of RmaxC (104).

Ⓛ Dental X-ray: radiological signs compatible with stage 5 tooth resorption in the upper incisor teeth.

Ⓜ Dental X-ray: artefact.

Ⓝ Dental X-ray: (from right to left) radiological signs compatible with vertical bone loss in LmandM1 (309) and LmandP4 (308).

Ⓞ Dental X-ray: radiological signs compatible with stage 4 periodontal disease in LmandP4 (308) and LmandM1 (309), with class 3 furcation.

Ⓟ Dental X-ray: radiological signs compatible with stage 2 tooth resorption in LmandP4 (308) and LmandM1 (309).

Ⓠ Dental X-ray: radiological signs compatible with stage 5 tooth resorption in LmandP3 (307).

Key diagnostic/treatment points

Periodontal disease is the most frequent oral disease in cats. Each tooth must be assessed and its corresponding stage of periodontal disease must be determined. A high stage of periodontal disease does not always correspond with a high gingival, bacterial plaque or dental calculus index. The definitive oral examination by means of a periodontal probe and dental X-rays will give us the information needed for a true assessment of the status of the disease in each tooth. Pathologies such as tooth resorption, though unrelated, can also be detected in the same patient in different teeth and at different stages.

Common errors

Determining the stage of periodontal disease of a tooth by its macroscopic state, without performing any complementary testing such as periodontal probing and/or dental radiology.

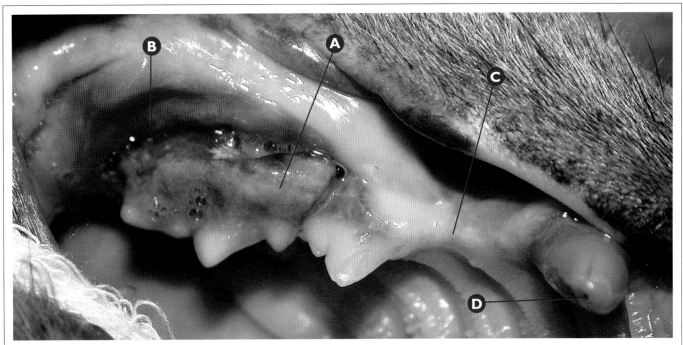

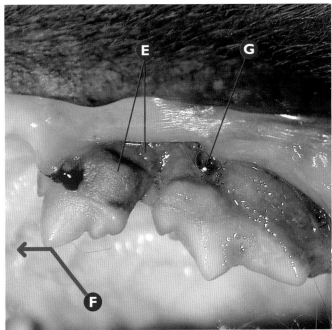

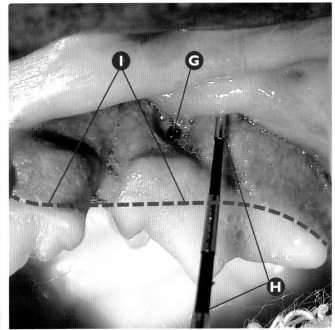

Bacterial, viral, fungal and parasitic origin | **Periodontal disease**

Suspected stage 4 periodontal disease in RmaxP4 (108), LmaxP3 (207) and LmaxP4 (208).

Ⓐ Calculus index 4 on RmaxP4 (108).

Ⓑ Gingival index 3 in RmaxP4 (108).

Ⓒ Absence of RmaxP2 (106).

Ⓓ Suspicions of a complicated crown fracture of RmaxC (104).

Ⓔ Severe build-up of dental calculus on the distal root of LmaxP3 (207).

Ⓕ Mesial displacement of LmaxP3 (207), likely caused by stage 4 periodontal disease.

Ⓖ Suspected class 3 furcation in LmaxP4 (208).

Ⓗ Upper probing depth greater than 6 mm in the vestibular area of LmaxP4 (208), determined using a periodontal probe.

Ⓘ Virtual line of the regional physiological gingival margin.

Key diagnostic/treatment points
Periodontal disease is the most frequent oral disease in cats. The different stages of periodontal disease should be individually assessed in each tooth. In this clinical case, we suspected stage 4 periodontal disease in various teeth, with different clinical signs. The confirmation of this stage must be done by means of complete probing of the affected teeth, as well as by dental X-rays.

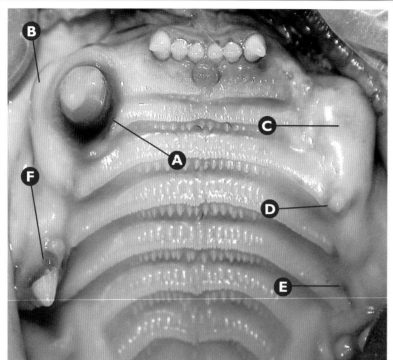

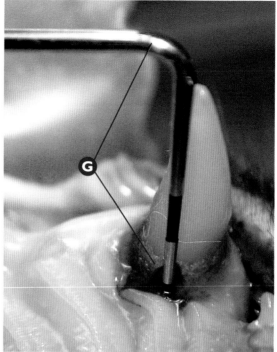

Bacterial, viral, fungal and parasitic origin | Periodontal disease

Stage 4 periodontal disease in RmaxC (104).

Ⓐ Suspected stage 4 periodontal disease in RmaxC (104).

Ⓑ Suspicions of expansion of the vestibular bone, typical in advanced stages of periodontal disease in the upper canine teeth of cats.

Ⓒ Absence of LmaxC (204).

Ⓓ LmaxP2 (206).

Ⓔ Absence of LmaxP3 (207).

Ⓕ Suspicions of tooth resorption in RmaxP3 (107).

Ⓖ Confirmation of stage 4 periodontal disease measured using a periodontal probe in the palatal area of RmaxC (104); periodontal pocket greater than 6 mm.

Ⓗ Dental X-ray: radiological signs compatible with expansion of the vestibular bone in RmaxC (104).

Ⓘ Dental X-ray: radiological signs compatible with stage 4 periodontal disease in RmaxC (104).

Ⓙ Dental X-ray: radiological signs compatible with root resorption of RmaxC (104).

Ⓚ Dental X-ray: radiological signs compatible with a root fragment of LmaxC (204).

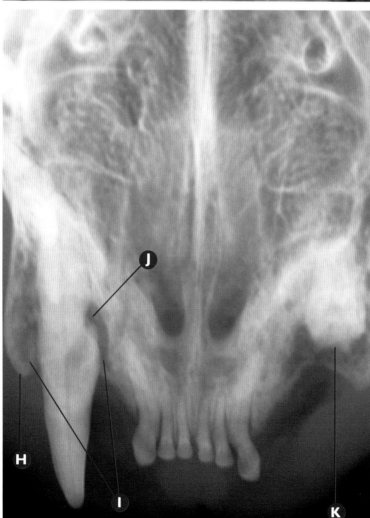

Key diagnostic/treatment points
Periodontal probing is fundamental together with dental X-rays to assess the stages of periodontal disease in cats. Two abnormalities that are uncommon in dogs are typically detected in the upper canine teeth of cats in the advanced stages of the disease: on the one hand, expansion of the vestibular bone, which is usually detected with deep periodontal pockets (present in this clinical case); and on the other hand, dental extrusion (abnormality detected frequently).

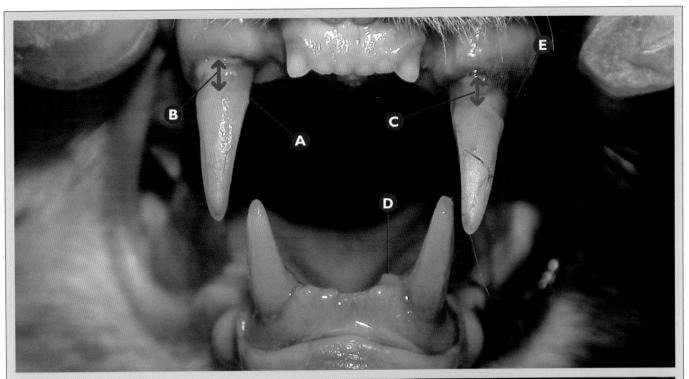

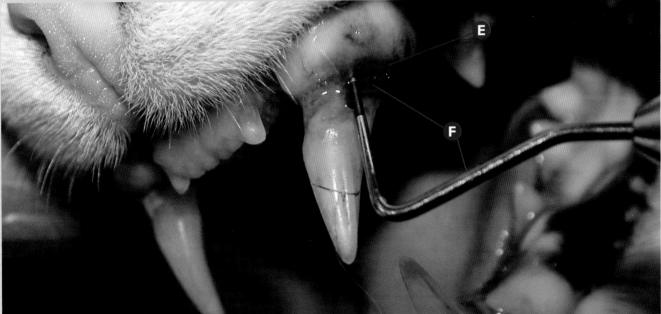

Suspected stage 4 periodontal disease in RmaxC (104) and LmaxC (204), with moderate extrusion.

Ⓐ Area of the cementoenamel junction of RmaxC (104).

Ⓑ Extrusion of RmaxC (104) outside the dental alveolus.

Ⓒ Extrusion of LmaxC (204) outside the dental alveolus.

Ⓓ Lingual deviation of Lmandl3 (303).

Ⓔ Gingival index 3 in LmaxC (204).

Ⓕ Confirmation, by means of periodontal probing, of stage 4 periodontal disease in LmaxC (204), with a probing depth greater than 9 mm in the vestibular area of LmaxC (204).

Key diagnostic/treatment points

While it is uncommon in dogs, in many cases of advanced stages of periodontal disease in the upper canine teeth of cats, canine tooth extrusion occurs, thus giving the appearance that the "fangs have grown" as many clients seem to claim. After confirmation of the disease by means of a regional dental radiological study, any teeth with stage 4 periodontal disease should be extracted.

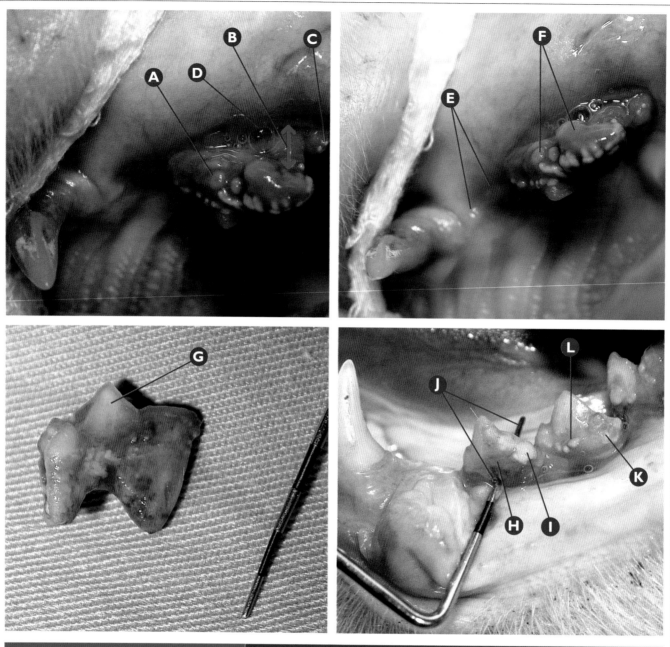

Bacterial, viral, fungal and parasitic origin | **Periodontal disease**

Stage 4 periodontal disease in LmaxP4 (208), and LmandP3 (307).

A Calculus index 4 on LmaxP4 (208).

B Exposure of the coronal third of the distal root of LmaxP4 (208), covered by calculus.

C Calculus index 4 on LmaxM1 (209).

D Gingival index 3 in LmaxP4 (208).

E Absence of LmaxP2 (206) and LmaxP3 (207).

F Close-up of calculus index 4 on LmaxP4 (208).

G Close-up of LmaxP4 (208), after its extraction due to stage 4 periodontal disease.

H Plaque index 2 on LmandP3 (307).

I Calculus index 2 on LmandP3 (307).

J Class 3 furcation in LmandP3 (307).

K Plaque index 2 on LmandP4 (308).

L Calculus index 2 on LmandP4 (308).

Key diagnostic/treatment points

Bacterial plaque and dental calculus indices, in spite of being closely related to periodontal disease, do not always provide information about the stage of said disease. In the case of LmaxP4 (208), the high dental calculus index corresponds with stage 4 periodontal disease. In the case of LmandP3 (307), periodontal disease is classified as stage 4 because of the class 3 furcation, although the tooth has low bacterial plaque and dental calculus indices. The confirmation of the stage of periodontal disease must be done using dental X-rays.

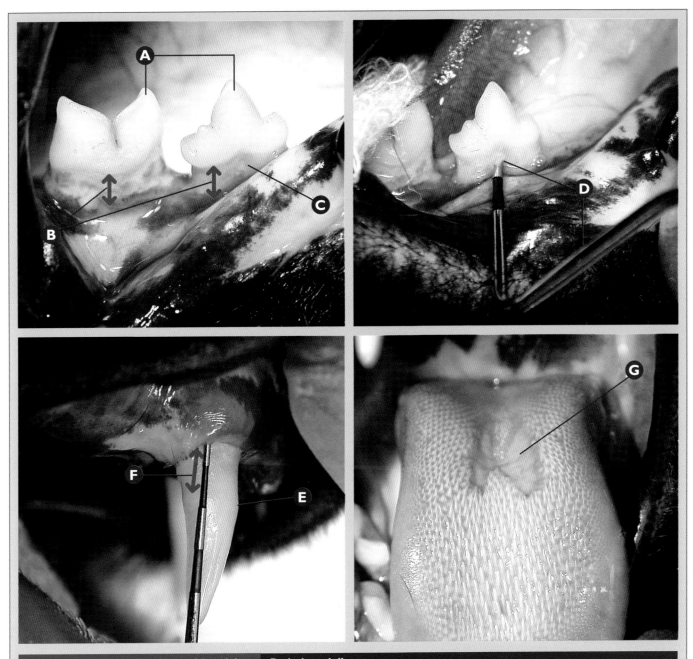

Stage 4 periodontal disease in RmandP4 (408).

A From right to left: RmandP4 (408) and RmandM1 (409).

B Areas of gingival retraction in RmandP4 (408) and RmandM1 (409).

C Suspected stage 4 periodontal disease in RmandP4 (408), with class 3 furcation.

D Confirmation of stage 4 periodontal disease in RmandP4 (408), with class 3 furcation.

E Area of the cementoenamel junction of RmaxC (104).

F 5-mm extrusion of RmaxC (104).

G Chronic ulcer on the dorsal surface of the tongue.

Key diagnostic/treatment points

In those cases where there is reasonable doubt regarding the stage of periodontal disease, it can be confirmed simply by means of periodontal probing using a dental probe. In the case of RmandP4 (408), stage 4 periodontal disease is confirmed by the presence of a class 3 furcation. This tooth must be extracted.

The appearance of ulcers on the dorsal surface of the tongue is relatively frequent, with many possible aetiologies that go from trauma to viral causes.

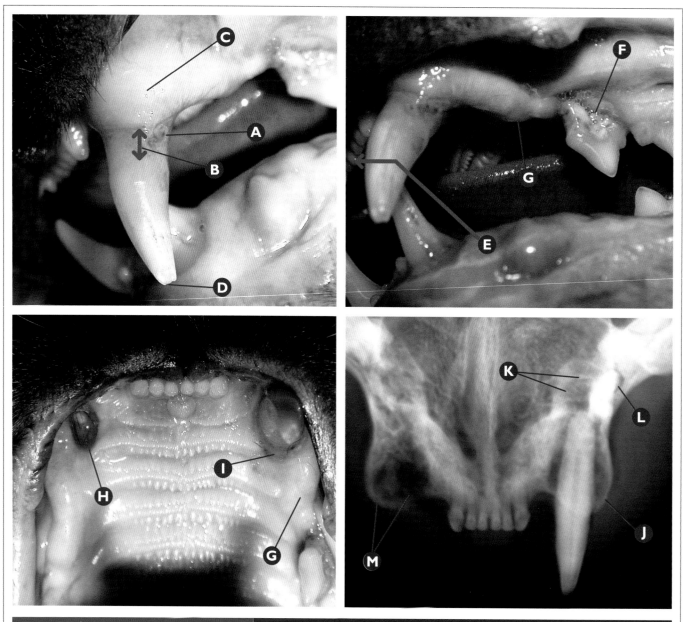

Stage 4 periodontal disease in LmaxC (204).

A Suspected stage 4 periodontal disease in RmaxC (204).

B Extrusion of LmaxC (204), due to periodontal disease.

C Thickening of the mucosa due to buccal bone expansion in LmaxC (204).

D Suspicions of fractured enamel on LmaxC (204).

E Mesial displacement of LmaxC (204), due to class 3 mobility.

F Stage 4 periodontal disease in LmaxP3 (207).

G Absence of LmaxP2 (206).

H Suspicions of absence of RmaxC (104) without complete closure of the wound, with the alveolus exposed.

I Drainage of purulent fluid in the subgingival area of LmaxC (204).

J Dental X-ray: radiological signs compatible with severe expansion of the vestibular bone in LmaxC (204).

K Dental X-ray: radiological signs compatible with periapical pathology of LmaxC (204).

L Dental X-ray: radiological signs compatible with periapical granuloma of the distal root of LmaxP3 (207).

M Dental X-ray: radiological signs compatible with absence of RmaxC (104), with regional bone expansion.

Key diagnostic/treatment points
When a tooth loses its bone insertion due to severe changes to the periodontal ligament, as occurs in LmaxC (204) in this clinical case, the tooth may have a high degree of mobility, leading to the eventual loss of the tooth. Advanced periodontal disease is also the most probable cause of the absence of RmaxC (104). Treatment of stage 4 periodontal disease in LmaxC (204) is dental extraction.

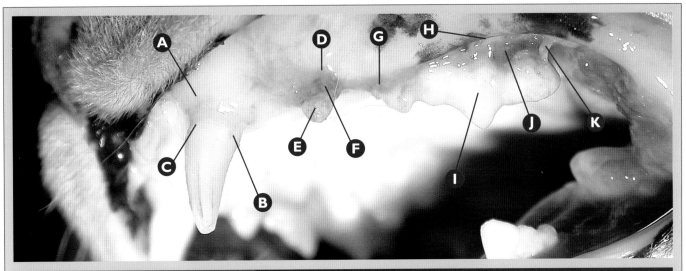

Bacterial, viral, fungal and parasitic origin   **Periodontal disease**

Suspected stage 1 to 3 periodontal disease in different teeth.

A Suspected stage 1 periodontal disease in LmaxC (204).

B Calculus index 1 on LmaxC (204).

C Plaque index 3 on LmaxC (204).

D Suspected stage 2 periodontal disease in LmaxP2 (206).

E Calculus index 2 on LmaxP2 (206).

F Gingival index 3 in LmaxP2 (206).

G Suspicions of a complicated crown-root fracture of LmaxP3 (207).

H Suspected stage 3 periodontal disease in LmaxP4 (208).

I Plaque index 4 on LmaxP4 (208).

J Gingival index 3 in LmaxP4 (208).

K Mucopurulent saliva on the surface of the crown of LmaxP4 (208).

Key diagnostic/treatment points

The plaque and dental calculus and gingival indices are merely informative, not definitive, for the assessment of the stage of periodontal disease. To adequately assess the stage of periodontal disease, we must use a periodontal probe and perform a dental radiological diagnosis.

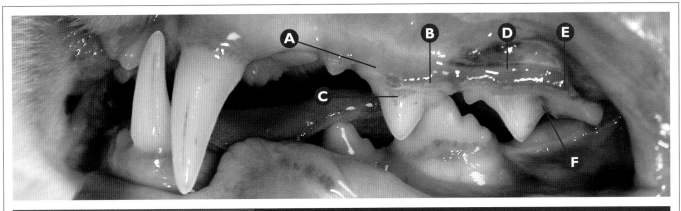

Bacterial, viral, fungal and parasitic origin   **Periodontal disease**

Stage 1 periodontal disease in LmaxP3 (207), and LmaxP4 (208).

A Stage 1 periodontal disease in LmaxP3 (207).

B Gingival index 1 in LmaxP3 (207).

C Calculus index 1 on LmaxP3 (207).

D Stage 1 periodontal disease in LmaxP4 (208).

E Gingival index 2 in LmaxP4 (208).

F Calculus index 2 on LmaxP4 (208).

Key diagnostic/treatment points

Mild stages of periodontal disease are reversible in many clinical cases. Adequate routine periodontal treatment (teeth cleaning) as well as the maintenance of oral hygiene once the animal is at home helps ensure proper oral health.

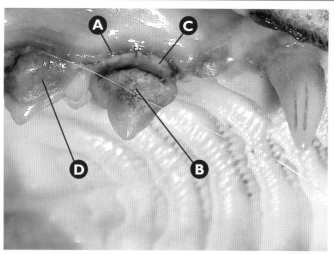

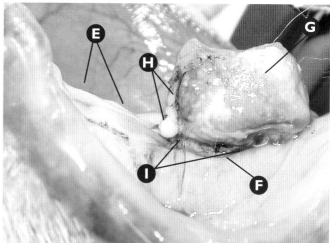

Bacterial, viral, fungal and parasitic origin | **Periodontal disease**

Suspected stage 4 periodontal disease in RmaxP3 (107), and LmandM1 (309).

Ⓐ Suspected stage 4 periodontal disease in RmaxP3 (107).

Ⓑ Calculus index 4 on RmaxP3 (107).

Ⓒ Accumulation of bacterial plaque with pus in the gingival region.

Ⓓ Calculus index 3 on RmaxP4 (108).

Ⓔ From right to left: absence of RmandP4 (308) and LmandP3 (307).

Ⓕ Suspected stage 4 periodontal disease in LmandM1 (309).

Ⓖ Calculus index 4 on LmandM1 (309).

Ⓗ Pus on the surface of the crown and covering the dental calculus.

Ⓘ Drainage of serosanguinolent fluid on the affected gingival margin.

Key diagnostic/treatment points
In spite of the visible calculus index, as well as the clear signs compatible with advanced periodontal disease, the exact stage of the disease should be confirmed by means of probing depths and dental X-rays.

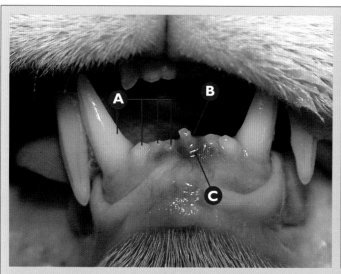

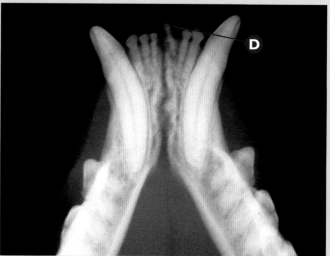

Bacterial, viral, fungal and parasitic origin | **Periodontal disease**

Stage 4 periodontal disease in LmandI1 (301).

Ⓐ From right to left: RmandI1 (401), RmandI2 (402), RmandI3 (403), RmandC (404).

Ⓑ Suspected stage 4 periodontal disease in LmandI1 (301), due to extrusion of the tooth.

Ⓒ Gingival index 3 in LmandI1 (301).

Ⓓ Dental X-ray: radiological signs compatible with stage 4 periodontal disease in LmandI1 (301).

Key diagnostic/treatment points
Occasionally, we can detect teeth with an advanced stage of periodontal disease, without it significantly affecting the surrounding teeth at that moment. In this clinical case, the stage 4 periodontal disease requires dental extraction to avoid progress of the disease to the regional teeth.

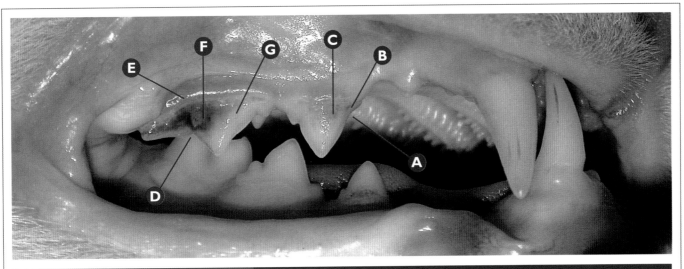

Bacterial, viral, fungal and parasitic origin   Periodontal disease

Stage 1 periodontal disease in RmaxP3 (107), and RmaxP4 (108).

Ⓐ Stage 1 periodontal disease in RmaxP3 (107).

Ⓑ Calculus index 1 on RmaxP3 (107).

Ⓒ Plaque index 2 on RmaxP3 (107).

Ⓓ Stage 1 periodontal disease in RmaxP4 (108).

Ⓔ Gingival index 1 in RmaxP4 (108).

Ⓕ Calculus index 2 on RmaxP4 (108).

Ⓖ Plaque index 2 on RmaxP4 (108).

Key diagnostic/treatment points
In some clinical cases, the dental calculus may take on different colours (from yellowish to dark brown, and including orange as seen here in this clinical case) that could be related to the composition of the saliva and the type and ingredients in the animal's food. This is when we should recommend periodontal treatment, given that we are generally faced with reversible situations that, over time, if adequate treatment measures are not taken, will become irreversible.

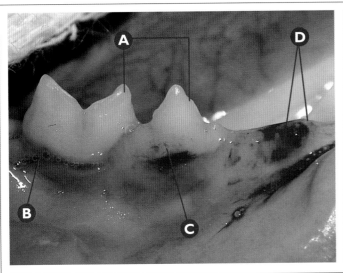
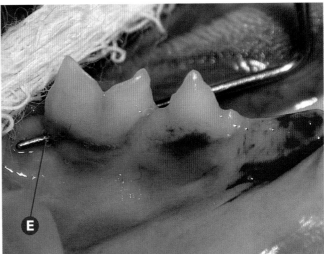

Bacterial, viral, fungal and parasitic origin   Periodontal disease

Suspected stage 4 periodontal disease in RmandM1 (409).

Ⓐ From right to left: RmandP4 (408), RmandM1 (409).

Ⓑ Suspected stage 2 periodontal disease in RmandM1 (409).

Ⓒ Suspected stage 2 tooth resorption in RmandP4 (408).

Ⓓ Absence of RmandP3 (407) with suspected stage 4b tooth resorption.

Ⓔ Stage 4 periodontal disease in RmandM1 (409), with class 3 furcation, confirmed by periodontal probing.

Key diagnostic/treatment points
The use of the probe and dental explorer is decisive to assess the stage of periodontal disease in some cases, even before performing dental X-rays. The latter will be especially useful in this clinical case to determine if RmandM1 (409) is affected by tooth resorption. Adequate treatment of RmandM1 (409) with class 3 furcation is dental extraction.

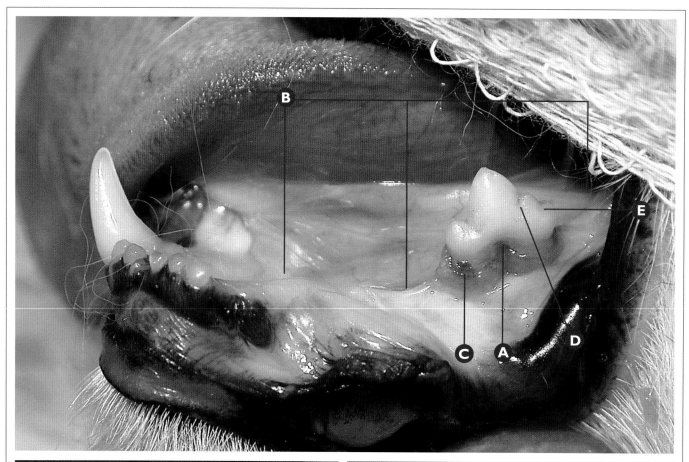

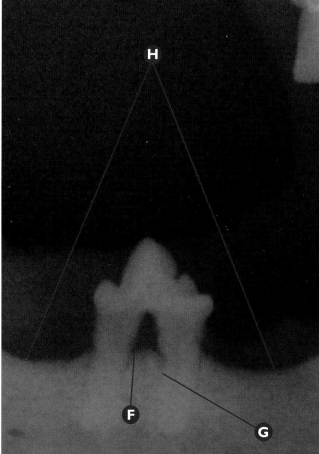

Periodontal disease

Stage 4 periodontal disease in LmandP4 (308).

Ⓐ Suspected stage 4 periodontal disease in RmandP4 (308).

Ⓑ From right to left: absence of LmandM1 (309), LmandP3 (307), LmandC (304).

Ⓒ Gingival index 2 in LmandP4 (308).

Ⓓ Plaque index 1 on LmandP4 (308).

Ⓔ Calculus index 0 on LmandP4 (308).

Ⓕ Dental X-ray: radiological signs compatible with stage 4 periodontal disease in LmandP4 (308), with class 3 furcation.

Ⓖ Dental X-ray: radiological signs compatible with stage 2 tooth resorption in LmandP4 (308).

Ⓗ Dental X-ray: (From right to left) radiological signs compatible with absence of LmandM1 (309) and LmandP3 (307).

Key diagnostic/treatment points

Aside from using a periodontal probe, furcation lesion classes may also be detected by regional dental X-rays. In this clinical case, radiographic detection of the exposure of the furcation area demonstrates the presence of stage 4 periodontal disease in LmandP4 (308).

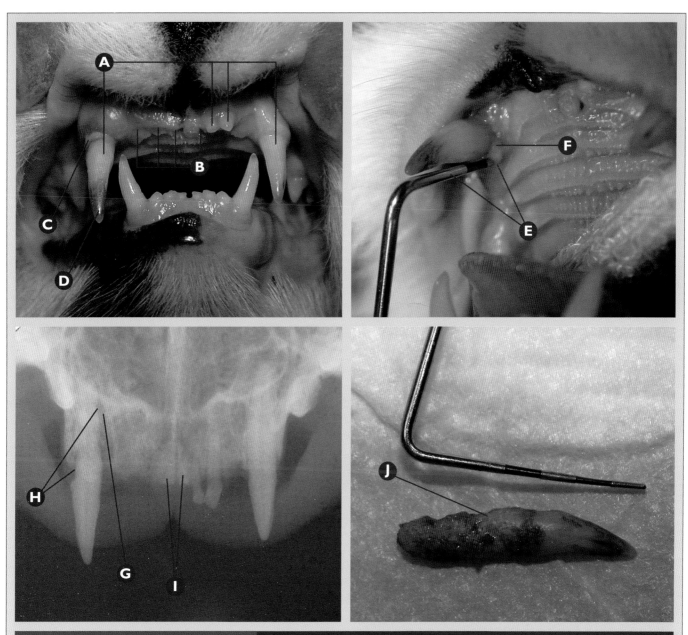

Stage 4 periodontal disease in RmaxC (104); dental discolouration due to a suspected type II endo-periodontal lesion.

Ⓐ From right to left: LmaxC (204), LmaxI3 (203), LmaxI2 (202) and RmaxC (104).

Ⓑ From right to left: absence of LmaxI1 (201), RmaxI1 (101), RmaxI2 (102) and RmaxI3 (103).

Ⓒ Suspected stage 3 periodontal disease in RmaxC (104).

Ⓓ Dental discolouration in the coronal third of the crown of RmaxC (104).

Ⓔ Confirmation of stage 4 periodontal disease in RmaxC (104), assessed using a periodontal probe in the palatal area of RmaxC (104); periodontal pocket of 8 mm.

Ⓕ Drainage of subgingival pus.

Ⓖ Dental X-ray: radiological signs compatible with stage 4 periodontal disease in RmaxC (104), due to loss of the periodontal ligament.

Ⓗ Dental X-ray: radiological signs compatible with stage 2 tooth resorption in RmaxC (104).

Ⓘ Dental X-ray: (from right to left) radiological signs compatible with stage 4b tooth resorption in LmaxI1 (201) and RmaxI1 (101).

Ⓙ Close-up of RmaxC (104), after its surgical extraction.

Key diagnostic/treatment points

Advanced stages of periodontal disease in the maxillary canine teeth will not always produce severe buccal bone expansion, or its macroscopic manifestation. We should always base the identification of the stage of periodontitis on the periodontal probing depth and dental X-rays. Occasionally, as in this clinical case, we can detect dental discolourations that are closely related to pulp pathologies (type II endo-periodontal lesion). Adequate treatment in this clinical case is dental extraction.

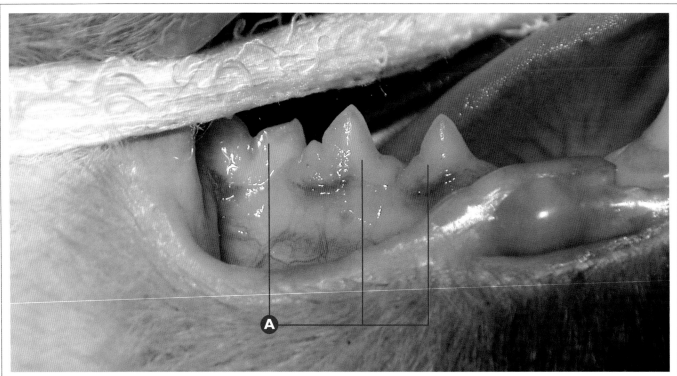

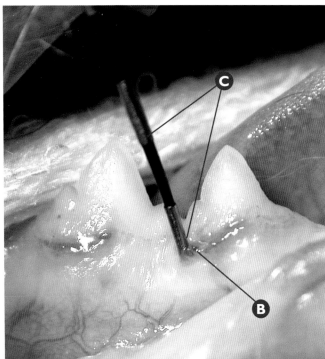

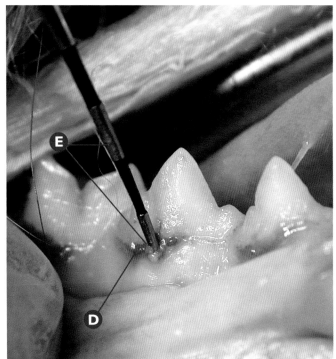

Bacterial, viral, fungal and parasitic origin | **Periodontal disease**

Suspected stage 1 periodontal disease in RmandP3 (407), and RmandP4 (408).

Ⓐ From right to left: RmandP3 (407), RmandP4 (408) and RmandM1(409).

Ⓑ Gingival index 1 in RmandP3 (407).

Ⓒ Gingival sulcus of 1 mm in the distovestibular area of RmandP3 (407), determined using a periodontal probe.

Ⓓ Gingival index 1 in RmandP4 (408).

Ⓔ Gingival sulcus of 1 mm in the vestibular area of RmandP4 (408), determined using a periodontal probe.

Key diagnostic/treatment points

We should recommend periodontal treatment (dental cleaning) when detecting these initial stages of periodontal disease. If no dental cleaning is performed, the progression will be evident, and the gingival indices and the stage of periodontitis will increase.

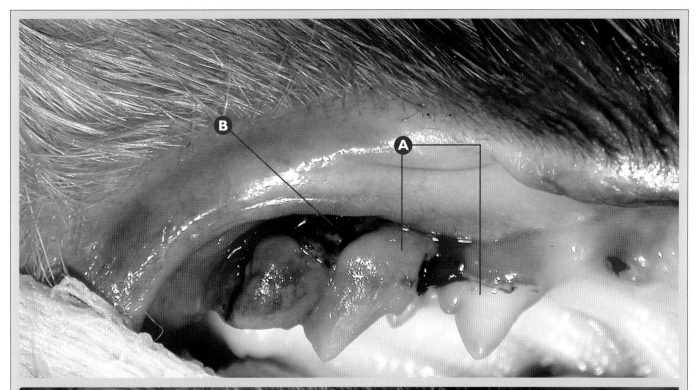

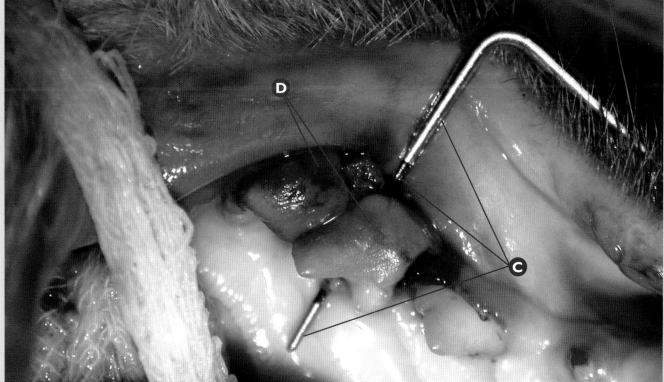

Stage 4 periodontal disease in RmaxP4 (108).

A From right to left: RmaxP3 (107) and RmaxP4 (108).

B Suspected stage 4 periodontal disease in RmaxP4 (108).

C Stage 4 periodontal disease in RmaxP4 (108), with class 3 furcation (confirmed by periodontal probing).

D Calculus index 4 on RmaxP4 (108).

Key diagnostic/treatment points

Once again, the use of the probe and dental explorer are fundamental to detect, and even occasionally classify, as in this clinical case, the stage of periodontal disease. The most appropriate treatment in this patient is the extraction of RmaxP4 (108).

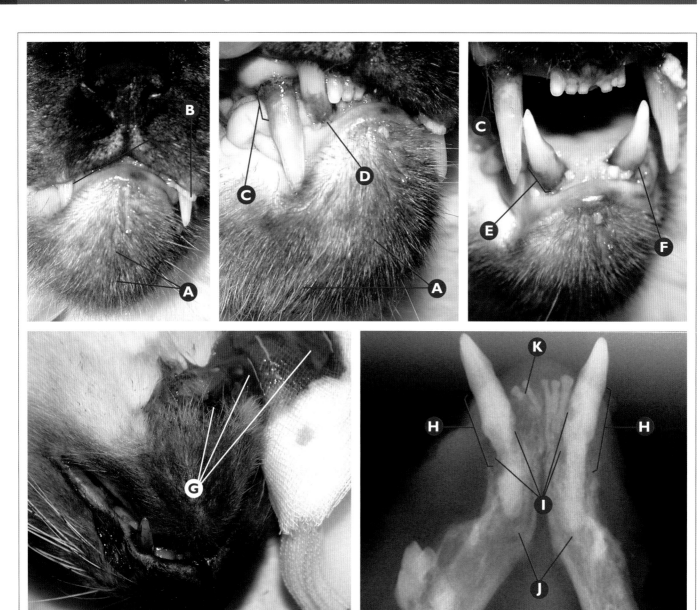

Bacterial, viral, fungal and parasitic origin   **Periodontal disease**

Stage 4 periodontal disease in LmandC (304) and RmandC (404), combined with a stage 3 tooth resorption in both teeth; formation of a severe periapical mandibular abscess.

A Severe mandibular abscess in the chin area.

B Visualisation of the cusps of the maxillary canine teeth outside the oral cavity, possible sign of advanced stage periodontal disease.

C Stage 4 periodontal disease in RmaxC (104).

D Suspected stage 4 periodontal disease in RmandC (404).

E Confirmation of stage 4 periodontal disease in RmandC (404).

F Suspected stage 4 periodontal disease in LmandC (304).

G Drainage of the severe mandibular abscess in the chin area with production of seropurulent fluid.

H Dental X-ray: (from right to left) radiological signs compatible with stage 4 periodontal disease in LmaxI1 (304) and RmaxI1 (404).

I Dental X-ray: (from right to left) radiological signs compatible with stage 3 tooth resorption in LmandC (304) and RmandC (404).

J Dental X-ray: radiological signs compatible with periapical pathology in LmandC (304) and RmandC (404).

K Dental X-ray: radiological signs compatible with stage 4c tooth resorption in RmandI2 (402).

Key diagnostic/treatment points

In advanced cases of periodontal disease in cats, extrusion of a tooth may occur, as seen in this clinical case in the maxillary and mandibular canine teeth. This stage of periodontal disease may single-handedly cause a periapical pathology that can develop into a dental abscess. This process may become complicated with the joint appearance of tooth resorption, which will accelerate the periapical pathology if it affects the pulp cavity. Treatment in this clinical case is the extraction of LmandC (304) and RmandC (404).

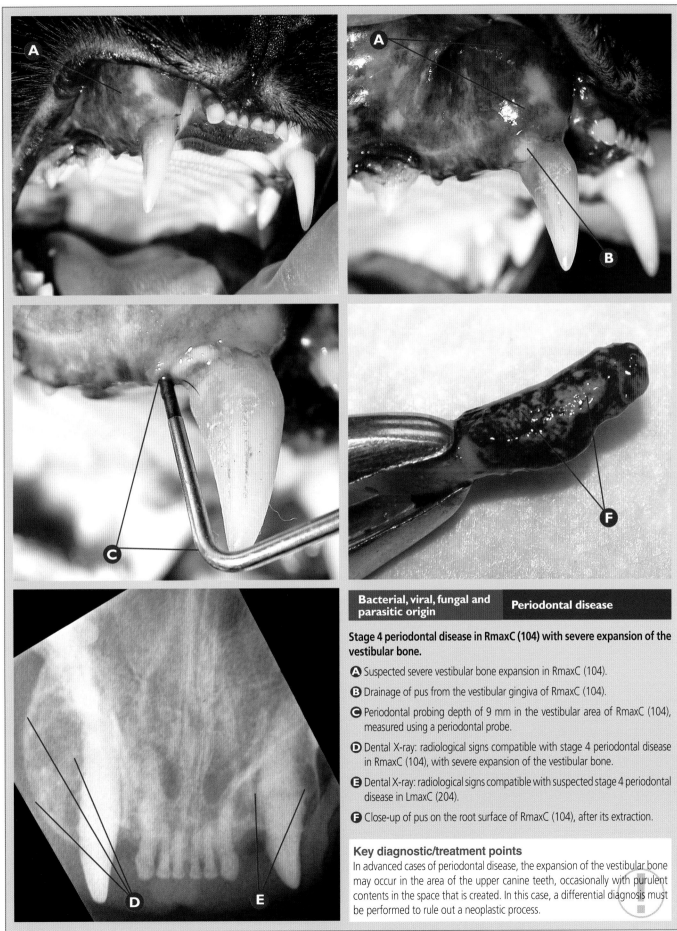

Bacterial, viral, fungal and parasitic origin | **Periodontal disease**

Stage 4 periodontal disease in RmaxC (104) with severe expansion of the vestibular bone.

Ⓐ Suspected severe vestibular bone expansion in RmaxC (104).

Ⓑ Drainage of pus from the vestibular gingiva of RmaxC (104).

Ⓒ Periodontal probing depth of 9 mm in the vestibular area of RmaxC (104), measured using a periodontal probe.

Ⓓ Dental X-ray: radiological signs compatible with stage 4 periodontal disease in RmaxC (104), with severe expansion of the vestibular bone.

Ⓔ Dental X-ray: radiological signs compatible with suspected stage 4 periodontal disease in LmaxC (204).

Ⓕ Close-up of pus on the root surface of RmaxC (104), after its extraction.

Key diagnostic/treatment points

In advanced cases of periodontal disease, the expansion of the vestibular bone may occur in the area of the upper canine teeth, occasionally with purulent contents in the space that is created. In this case, a differential diagnosis must be performed to rule out a neoplastic process.

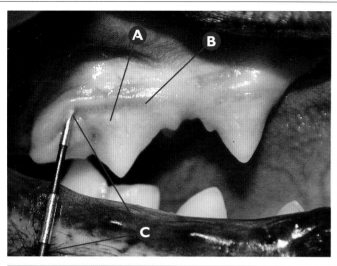
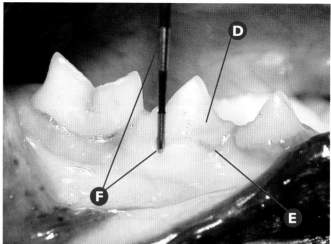

Bacterial, viral, fungal and parasitic origin | **Periodontal disease**

Suspected stage 1 periodontal disease in RmaxP4 (108), and RmandP4 (408).

Ⓐ Plaque index 3 on RmaxP4 (108).

Ⓑ Gingival index 1 in RmaxP4 (108).

Ⓒ Image of gingival sulcus probing using a periodontal probe in the vestibular area of RmaxP4 (108); sulcus depth is 1 mm.

Ⓓ Plaque index 1 on RmandP4 (408).

Ⓔ Gingival index 1 in RmandP4 (408).

Ⓕ Image of ginvigal sulcus probing using a periodontal probe in the vestibular area of RmandP4 (408); sulcus depth is less than 1 mm.

Key diagnostic/treatment points
In the initial stages of periodontal disease, we should provide our clients with recommendations on how to perform adequate oral hygiene for their cat; dental brushing with specific toothpaste must be the base of this maintenance of the hygiene.

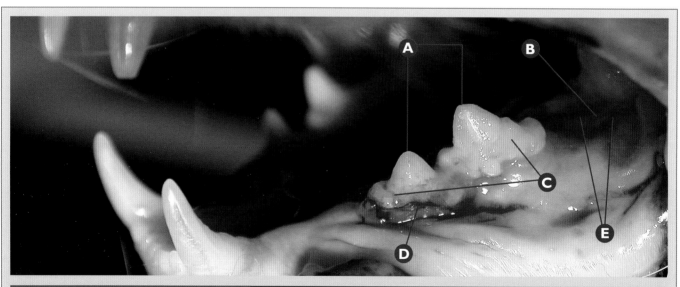

Bacterial, viral, fungal and parasitic origin | **Periodontal disease**

Suspected stage 2 periodontal disease in LmandP3 (307), and RmandP4 (308).

Ⓐ From right to left: LmandP4 (308) and LmandP3 (307).

Ⓑ Absence of LmandM1 (309).

Ⓒ Plaque index 3 on LmandP3 (307) and LmandP4 (308).

Ⓓ Gingival index 2 in LmandP3 (307).

Ⓔ Moderate-severe gingivostomatitis in the region of the absent LmandM1 (309).

Key diagnostic/treatment points
The control and elimination of bacterial plaque, by maintaining oral hygiene at home or by means of routine professional periodontal treatment, must be one of our primary objectives in the treatment of periodontal disease.

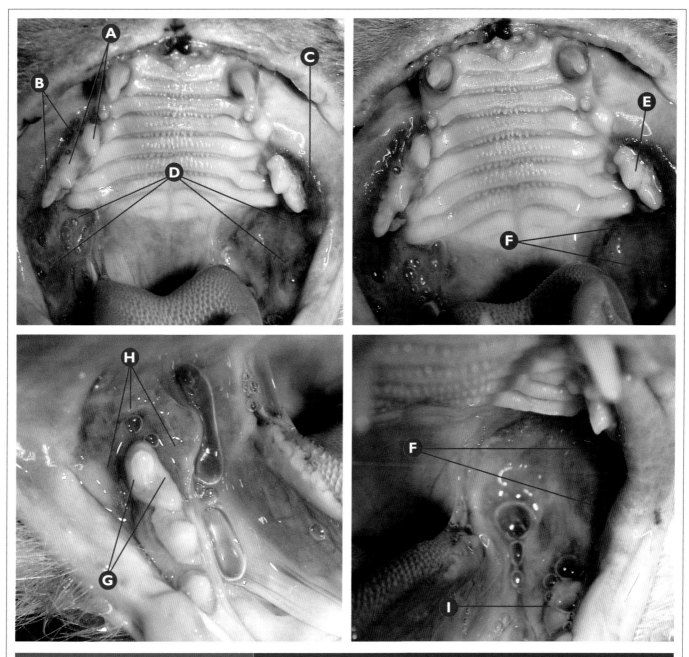

Severe chronic feline gingivostomatitis in an 11-year-old patient. Viral analysis (PCR): FeLV -, FIV -, FCV +, FHV -.

Ⓐ Plaque index 4 on RmaxP3 (107) and RmaxP4 (108).

Ⓑ Gingival index 3 in RmaxP3 (107) and RmaxP4 (108).

Ⓒ Gingival index 3 in LmaxP4 (208).

Ⓓ Severe stomatitis in the left and right caudal buccal mucosa.

Ⓔ Image of plaque index 4 on LmaxP4 (208).

Ⓕ Close-up of severe stomatitis in the left caudal buccal mucosa.

Ⓖ Plaque index 4 on RmandM1 (409).

Ⓗ Severe gingivostomatitis in the vestibular, distal and lingual regions of RmandM1 (409).

Ⓘ LmandM1 (309).

Key diagnostic/treatment points
Chronic feline gingivostomatitis is a very frequent pathology in daily feline clinical practice. Many studies have been conducted to determine its aetiology and how it should be treated. Periodontal disease and viral infections seem to be closely associated with this disease. The feline calicivirus may play a determinant role in this syndrome. Adequate viral detection and control of periodontal disease (including multiple extractions of premolars and molars if needed) are the first steps to follow to control this feline disease.

The general clinical signs and those detected in the oral cavity are highly variable; the clinical picture ranges from no evident signs to anorexia and severe oral pain, with a wide variety of clinical signs between the two extremes.

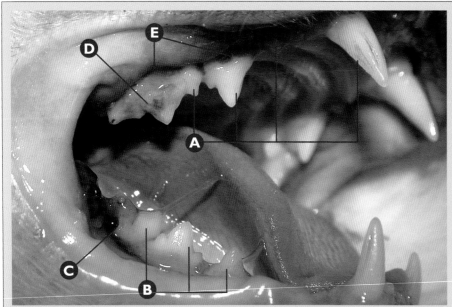

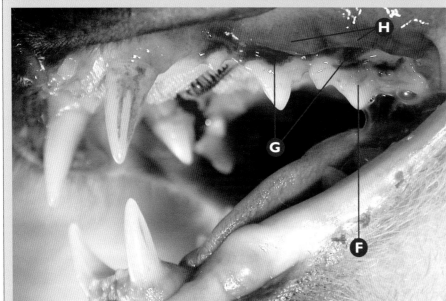

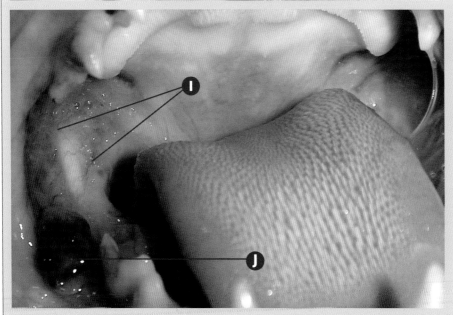

Bacterial, viral, fungal and parasitic origin
Feline gingivostomatitis

Moderate chronic feline gingivostomatitis in a 4-year-old patient; on long-term corticosteroid treatment.
Viral analysis (PCR): FeLV -, FIV -, FCV +, FHV -.

A From right to left: RmaxC (104), RmaxP2 (106), RmaxP3 (107) and RmaxP4 (108).

B From right to left: RmandP3 (407), RmandP4 (408) and RmandM1(409).

C Suspected class 3 tooth resorption in RmandM1 (409).

D Plaque index 4 on RmaxP4 (108).

E Gingival index 3 in RmaxP3 (107) and RmaxP4 (108).

F Plaque index 4 on LmaxP4 (208).

G Gingival index 3 in LmaxP3 (207) and LmaxP4 (208).

H Severe stomatitis in the vestibular region of LmaxP3 (207) and LmaxP4 (208).

I Moderate involvement of the right caudal buccal mucosa.

J Hyperplastic tissue in the vestibular region of RmandM1 (409).

Key diagnostic/treatment points
In this case of chronic feline gingivostomatitis, there is a gingival index 3 in the upper premolars (studies performed consider periodontal disease as one of the possible aetiologies involved), in spite of the animal being on long-term corticosteroid therapy. The administration of corticosteroids may explain the moderate involvement of the left and right caudal buccal mucosa. Control of the periodontal disease in this clinical case is necessary to treat the clinical signs.

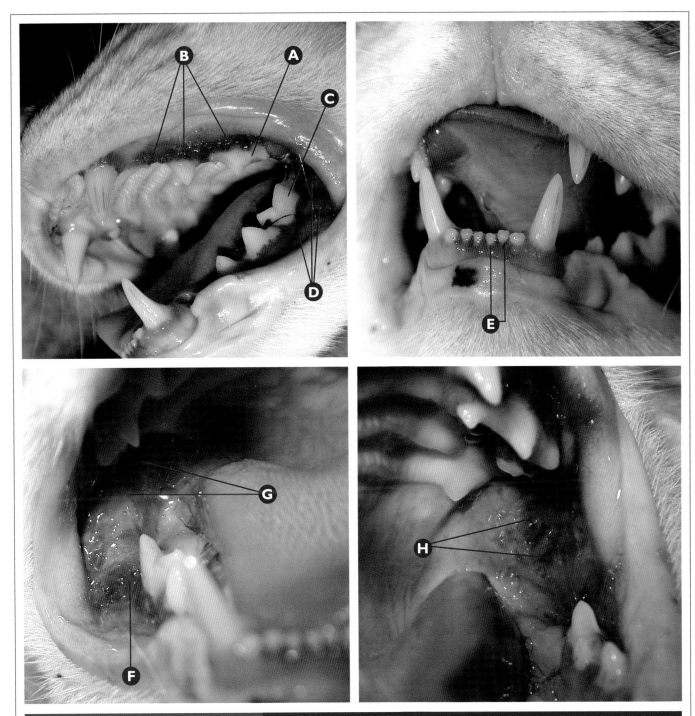

Bacterial, viral, fungal and parasitic origin | **Feline gingivostomatitis**

Severe chronic feline gingivostomatitis in a 13-month-old patient.
Viral analysis (PCR): FeLV -, FIV -, **FCV +**, FHV -.

Ⓐ Plaque index 4 on LmaxP4 (208).

Ⓑ Gingival index 3 in LmaxP2 (206), LmaxP3 (207) and LmaxP4 (208).

Ⓒ Plaque index 3 on LmandM1 (309).

Ⓓ Severe gingivostomatitis in the vestibular and distal regions of LmandM1 (309).

Ⓔ From right to left: gingival index 3 in LmandI2 (302) and LmandI1 (301).

Ⓕ Severe gingivostomatitis in the distal region of RmandM1 (409).

Ⓖ Moderate-severe stomatitis in the right caudal buccal mucosa.

Ⓗ Severe stomatitis in the left caudal buccal mucosa.

Key diagnostic/treatment points
Chronic feline gingivostomatitis is detected in those regions of the oral cavity that come into close contact with the teeth, in the caudal buccal mucosa or in the palatoglossal arch. If an incisional biopsy is viable, it is highly recommended to confirm the process, as well as viral detection in each case.

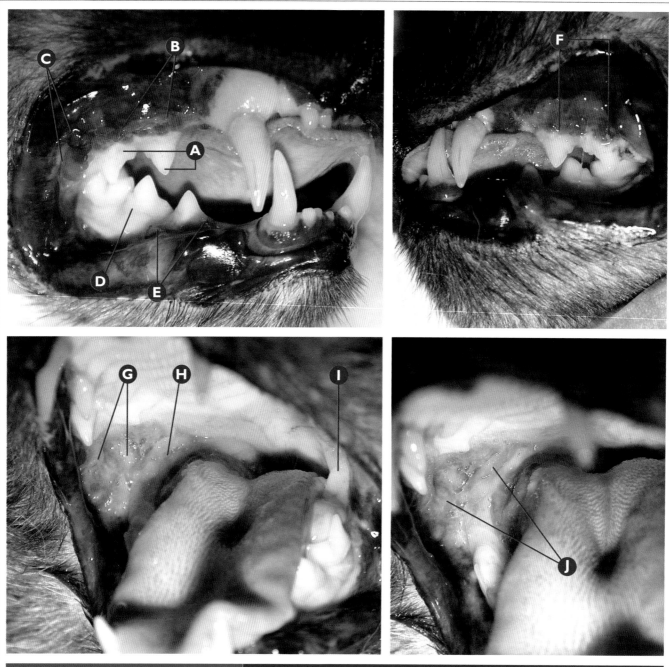

Bacterial, viral, fungal and parasitic origin | **Feline gingivostomatitis**

Severe chronic feline gingivostomatitis in an 11-year-old patient. Viral analysis (PCR): FeLV -, FIV -, **FCV +**, FHV -.

Ⓐ From right to left: index 3 of bacterial plaque on RmaxP3 (107) and RmaxP4 (108).

Ⓑ Gingival index 3 in RmaxP3 (107) and RmaxP4 (108).

Ⓒ Hyperplastic tissue in the mucosa in vestibular contact with RmaxP4 (108).

Ⓓ Gingival index 0 in RmandP4 (408).

Ⓔ Gingival index 3 in RmandP3 (407).

Ⓕ From right to left: gingival index 3 in LmaxP4 (208) and LmaxP3 (207).

Ⓖ Severe stomatitis in the right caudal buccal mucosa.

Ⓗ Moderate-severe stomatitis in the right palatoglossal arch.

Ⓘ Absence of stomatitis in the left palatoglossal arch.

Ⓙ Close-up of severe stomatitis in the right caudal buccal mucosa.

Key diagnostic/treatment points

Chronic gingivostomatitis, as can be seen in this clinical case, may affect the gingiva and mucosa in direct contact with the teeth as well as the caudal buccal mucosa and palatoglossal arch. In the latter two locations, it is not uncommon for one side to be more affected than the other, or there may be unilateral involvement without any obvious cause. In any case, this does not influence the general clinical picture, and numerous combinations between the oral and general clinical signs are possible.

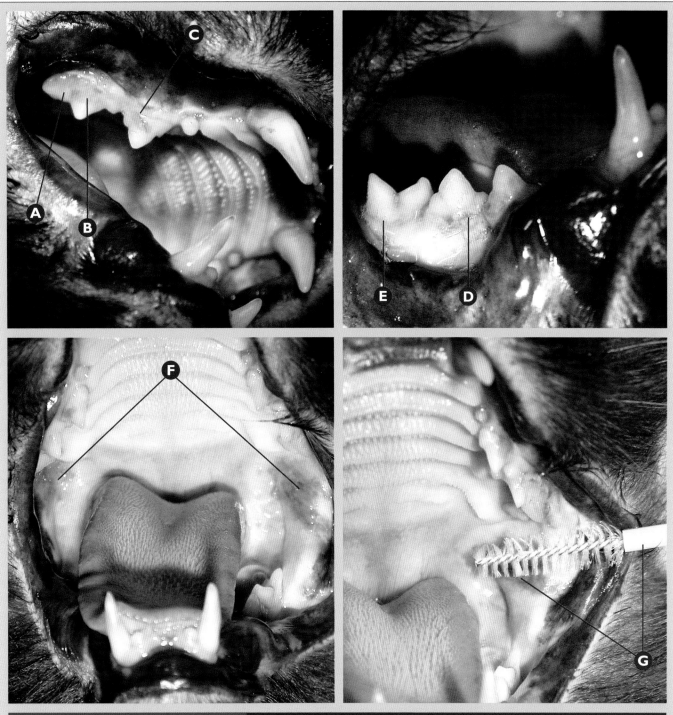

Bacterial, viral, fungal and parasitic origin | **Feline gingivostomatitis**

Mild chronic feline gingivostomatitis in a 5-year-old patient. Viral analysis (PCR): FeLV -, FIV -, **FCV +**, FHV -.

Ⓐ Plaque index 3 on RmaxP4 (108).

Ⓑ Calculus index 3 on RmaxP4 (108).

Ⓒ Gingival index 0 in RmaxP3 (107).

Ⓓ Gingival index 1 in RmandP4 (408).

Ⓔ Gingival index 0 in RmandM1 (409).

Ⓕ Mild stomatitis in the left and right caudal buccal mucosa.

Ⓖ Image of the cellular sample taken for PCR detection of FCV and FHV.

Key diagnostic/treatment points

In some cases of mild gingivostomatitis such as in this patient, we can also detect initial stages of periodontal disease. In this case, we can only detect a mild degree of stomatitis in both sides of the caudal buccal mucosa. A Cytobrush® can be used to collect oral mucosal cells to detect the presence of FCV (positive in this clinical case) and FHV (negative in this patient) by PCR.

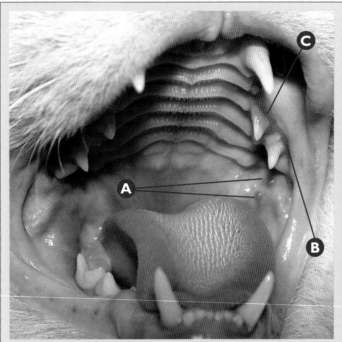
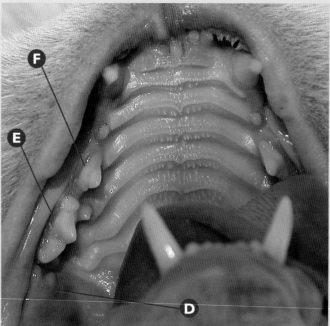
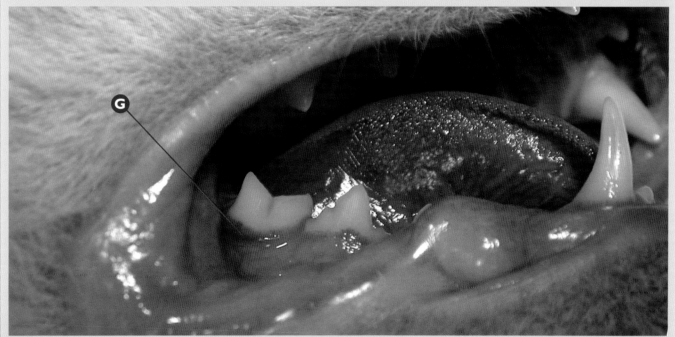

Bacterial, viral, fungal and parasitic origin | **Feline gingivostomatitis**

Mild chronic feline gingivostomatitis in a 10-month-old patient.
Viral analysis (PCR): FeLV -, FIV -, FCV +, FHV -.

A Mild stomatitis in the left caudal buccal mucosa.

B Gingival index 1 in LmaxP4 (208).

C Gingival index 1 in LmaxP3 (207).

D Mild stomatitis in the right caudal buccal mucosa, in the area distal to RmaxM1 (109).

E Gingival index 1 in RmaxP4 (108).

F Gingival index 1 in RmaxP3 (107).

G Gingival index 2 in RmandM1 (409).

Key diagnostic/treatment points

In some cases of mild gingivostomatitis with initial stages of periodontal disease, only mild gingivitis and stomatitis are detected in specific areas. Although in these cases there are no significant clinical signs, viral detection, control of the periodontitis, and monitoring of the progression of the oral and behavioural signs (appearance of pain signs) are recommended.

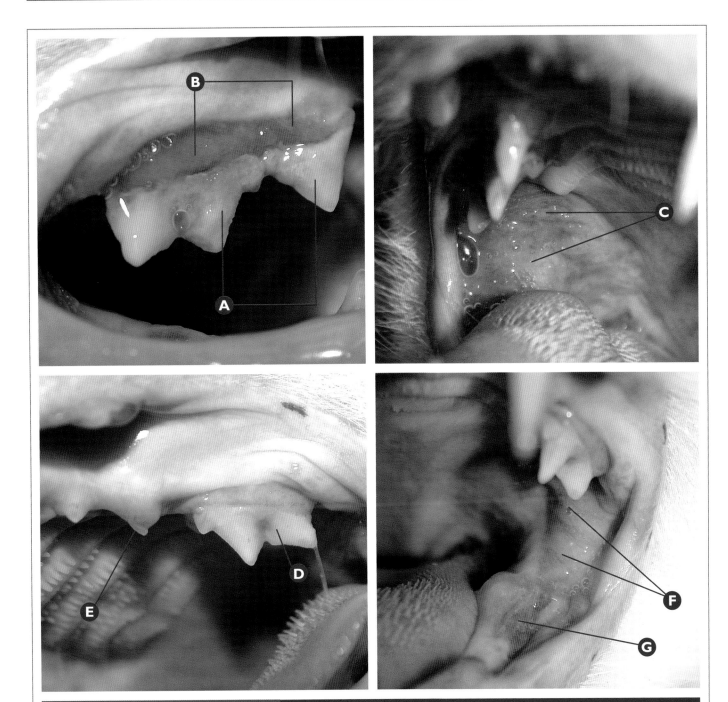

Bacterial, viral, fungal and parasitic origin   **Feline gingivostomatitis**

Moderate-severe chronic feline gingivostomatitis in an 8-year-old patient.
Viral analysis (PCR): FeLV -, FIV -, FCV +, FHV -.

Ⓐ From right to left: plaque index 4 on RmaxP3 (107) and RmaxP4 (108).

Ⓑ From right to left: gingival index 2 in RmaxP3 (107) and RmaxP4 (108).

Ⓒ Severe stomatitis in the right caudal buccal mucosa.

Ⓓ Plaque index 3 on LmaxP4 (208).

Ⓔ Suspected class 4 tooth resorption in LmaxP3 (207).

Ⓕ Moderate stomatitis in the left buccal caudal mucosa.

Ⓖ Suspicions of class 4b tooth resorption in LmandM1 (309), which is absent, with a possible root fragment and regional gingivitis.

Key diagnostic/treatment points

In numerous clinical cases of chronic gingivostomatitis, several teeth are affected by tooth resorption. Both diseases are not associated, although tooth resorption may worsen the clinical signs due to the greater deposition and accumulation of bacterial plaque (with the resulting appearance of gingivitis and regional stomatitis), and increase oral pain, which is common in patients affected by chronic feline gingivostomatitis.

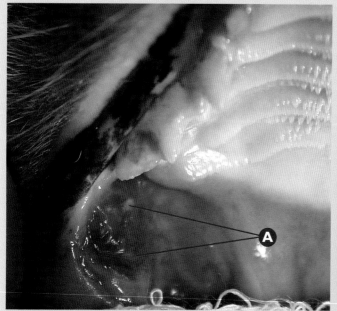

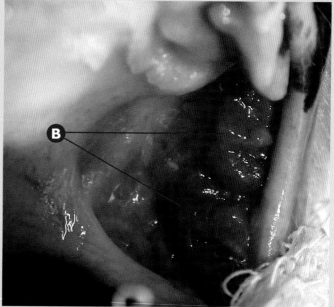

Bacterial, viral fungal and parasitic origin | Feline gingivostomatitis

Severe chronic feline gingivostomatitis in a 9-year-old patient. Viral analysis (PCR): FeLV -, FIV -, FCV +, FHV -.

(A) Severe stomatitis in the right caudal buccal mucosa.

(B) Severe stomatitis in the left caudal buccal mucosa with appearance of proliferative tissue.

(C) Postoperative follow-up after 21 days (periodontal treatment and multiple extractions of premolars and molars): adequate closure of the gingivae.

(D) Postoperative follow-up after 21 days: absence of stomatitis in the right caudal buccal mucosa.

(E) Postoperative follow-up after 21 days: absence of stomatitis in the left caudal buccal mucosa.

(F) Postoperative follow-up after 21 days: absence of stomatitis in the left caudal buccal mucosa.

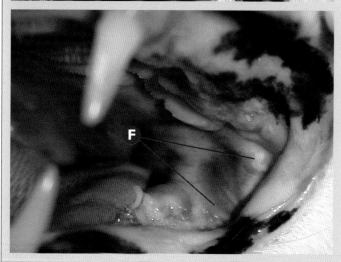

Key diagnostic/treatment points

A large body of literature describes multiple extractions of premolars and molars as a surgical treatment option for chronic feline gingivostomatitis, especially when oral pain is present. In this clinical case, the intervention allowed for the temporary resolution of the disease and its clinical signs (including in those areas where the formation of proliferative tissue had been detected); however, intensive monitoring is indicated.

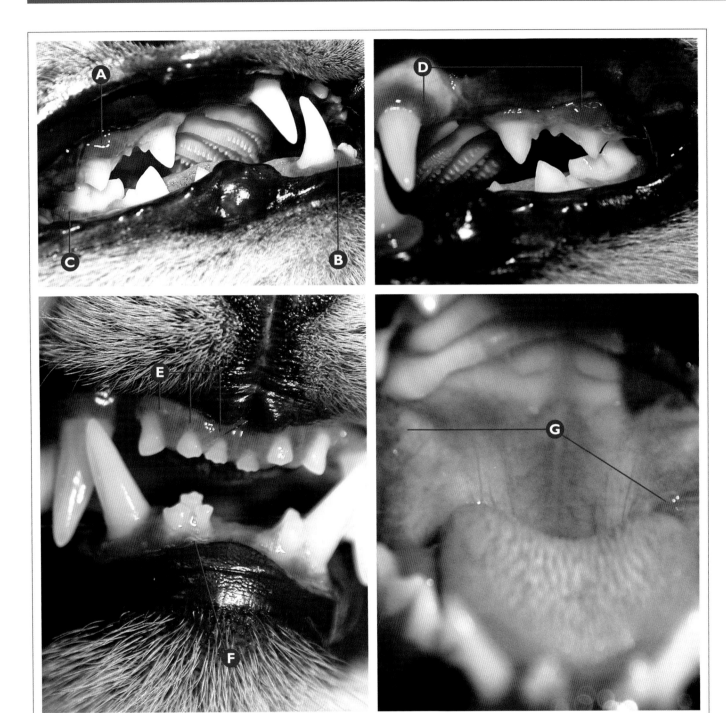

Bacterial, viral, fungal and parasitic origin | **Feline gingivostomatitis**

Moderate-severe chronic feline gingivostomatitis in an 8-month-old patient.
Viral analysis (PCR): FeLV -, FIV -, FCV +.

Ⓐ Gingival index 3 in RmaxP4 (108).

Ⓑ Gingival index 3 in RmandC (404).

Ⓒ Gingival index 3 in RmandM1 (409).

Ⓓ From right to left: gingival index 3 in LmaxP4 (208) and LmaxC (204).

Ⓔ From right to left: gingival index 2 in RmaxI1 (101), RmaxI2 (102) and RmaxI3 (103).

Ⓕ Suspected stage 4 periodontal disease in RmandI1 (401), RmandI2 (402) and RmandI3 (403).

Ⓖ Mild stomatitis in the right and left caudal buccal mucosa.

Key diagnostic/treatment points
Gingivostomatitis potentially associated with a viral infection can be detected even in young patients. In these cases, the deposition of bacterial plaque is not severe. However, these cases of gingivitis, as in this clinical case, can become very severe. In such young animals we should first suspect a viral cause and thus perform appropriate viral detection tests.

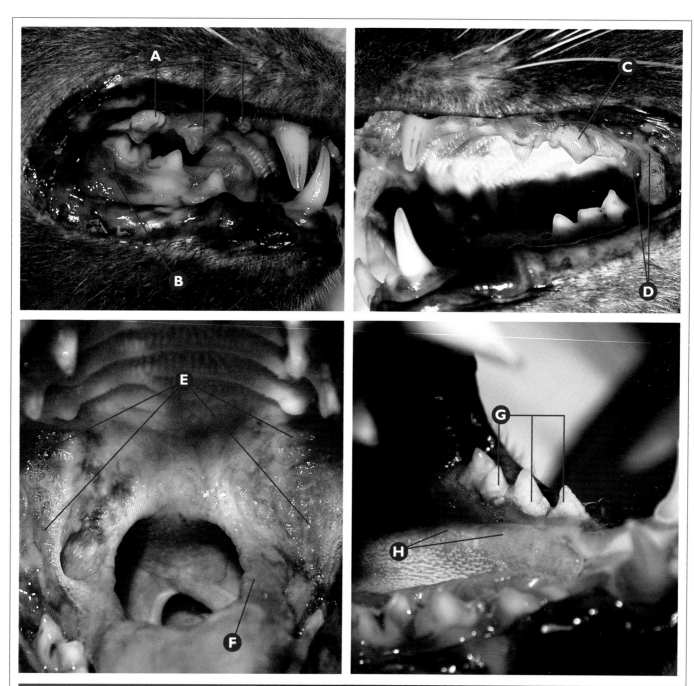

Bacterial, viral, fungal and parasitic origin   Feline gingivostomatitis

Moderate-severe chronic feline gingivostomatitis in an 18-year-old patient.
Viral analysis (PCR): FeLV -, FIV -, FCV +, FHV -.

Ⓐ From right to left: calculus index 4 on RmaxP2 (106), RmaxP3 (107) and RmaxP4 (108).

Ⓑ Proliferative tissue in the gingiva and mucosa in the vestibular area of RmandM1 (409).

Ⓒ Calculus index 4 on LmaxP4 (208).

Ⓓ Moderate-severe stomatitis in the left caudal buccal mucosa.

Ⓔ Severe stomatitis in the left and right caudal buccal mucosa.

Ⓕ Moderate stomatitis in the left palatoglossal arch.

Ⓖ From right to left: plaque index 4 on the lingual area of LmandP3 (307), LmandP4 (308) and LmandM1 (309).

Ⓗ Lesions in the left lateral margin of the tongue, due to contact with the bacterial plaque on the lingual surfaces of LmandP3 (307), LmandP4 (308) and LmandM1 (309).

Key diagnostic/treatment points
In cases of chronic gingivostomatitis, age is not a determinant factor when evaluating the diagnostic possibilities and treatment to improve the systemic and local oral signs. This 18-year-old patient suffers from calicivirus (FCV) and different stages of periodontal disease. The latter should definitely be treated.

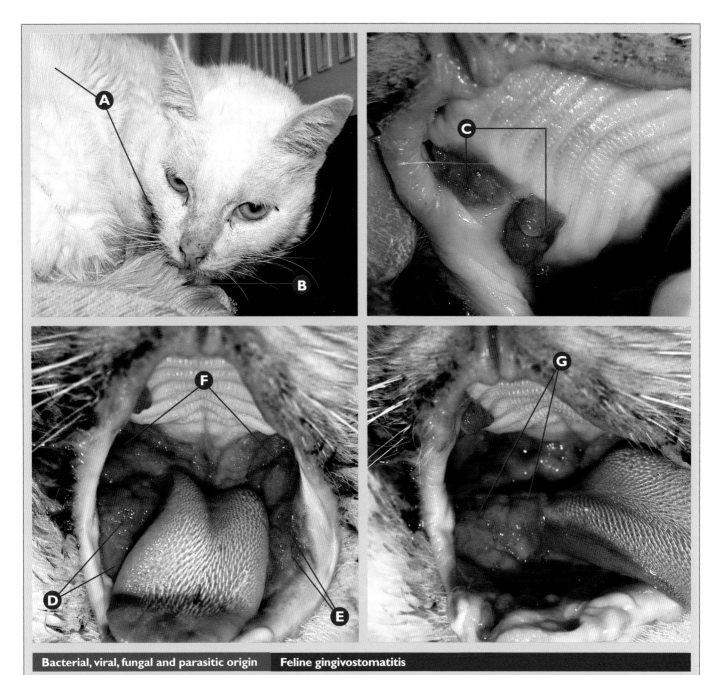

Bacterial, viral, fungal and parasitic origin | Feline gingivostomatitis

Severe chronic feline gingivostomatitis in a patient of unknown age.
Viral analysis (PCR): FeLV -, FIV -, FCV +, FHV -.

A Depressed patient due to chronic oral pain.

B Tip of the tongue protruding outside the oral cavity.

C From right to left: proliferative tissue, with severe gingivostomatitis in the area of RmaxP4 (108) and RmaxC (104) (both absent) (previous surgical extraction performed).

D Severe proliferative tissue with severe gingivostomatitis in the area of RmandP3 (407), RmandP4 (408) and RmandM1 (409) (all absent) (previous surgical extraction performed).

E Severe gingivostomatitis in the area of LmandP3 (307), LmandP4 (308) and LmandM1 (309) (all absent) (surgical extraction performed).

F Severe stomatitis in the left and right caudal buccal mucosa.

G Severe stomatitis with proliferative tissue in the right palatoglossal arch.

Key diagnostic/treatment points

In many cases of chronic feline gingivostomatitis, in spite of performing viral detection diagnostic tests and extensive surgical treatments recommended by several sources (such as multiple extractions of premolars and molars), and of administering different medical treatments (antibiotic therapy, steroid-based and non-steroid-based anti-inflammatory agents, immune modulators, antiviral agents, homoeopathy, etc.), the results of the management of this syndrome are not always satisfactory. Consequently, more specific diagnostic studies should be conducted, together with studies to identify adequate treatment options.

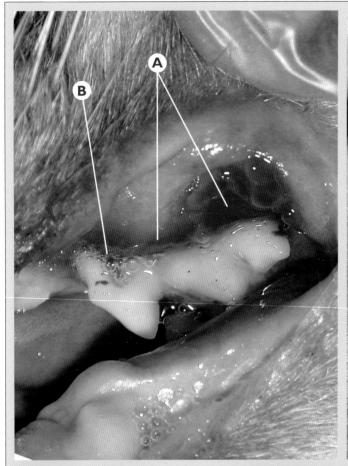

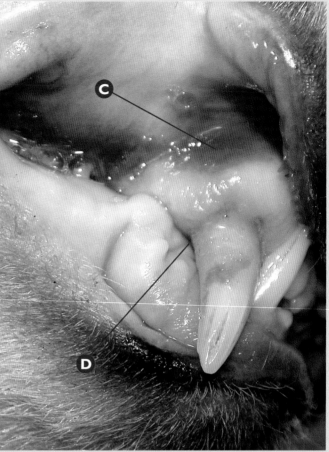

Bacterial, viral, fungal and parasitic origin | **Feline gingivostomatitis**

Severe chronic feline gingivostomatitis with severe lesions in the mucosa of the dorsal surface of the tongue.

Ⓐ Severe gingivostomatitis in the region of LmaxP3 (207) and LmaxP4 (208).

Ⓑ Stage 4 periodontal disease in LmaxP3 (207).

Ⓒ Severe stomatitis in the mucosa apical to RmaxC (104).

Ⓓ Suspected stage 4 periodontal disease in RmaxC (104).

Ⓔ Severe ulcer on the dorsal surface of the tongue.

Key diagnostic/treatment points

Ulcers detected on the tongue surface may be due to a calicivirus and/or feline herpes virus infection. The detection of these viruses and an adequate differential diagnosis should therefore be performed; other clinical signs that will confirm the suspicions of viral infection are likely to be detected in most of these patients. Any secondary infections must be properly treated and proper care of the animal must be ensured (hydration, correct and controlled feeding, etc.).

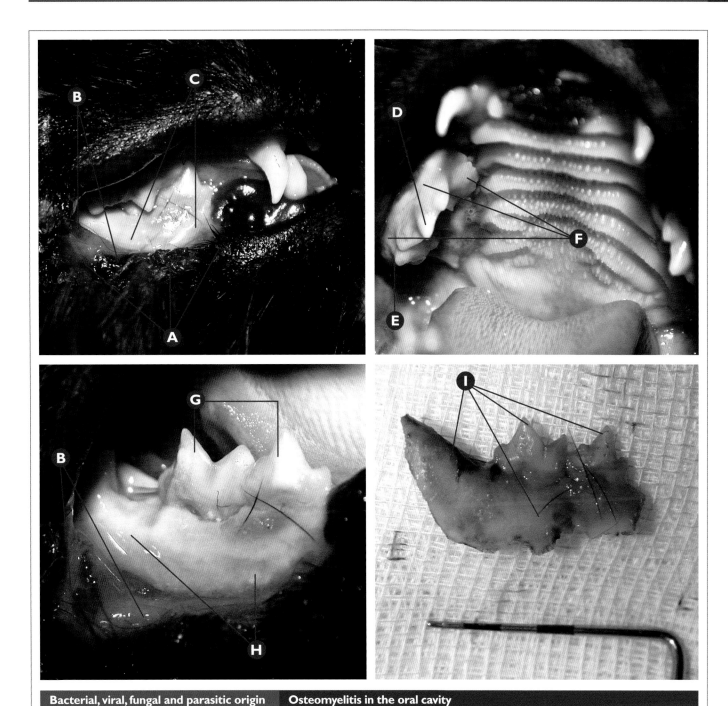

Bacterial, viral, fungal and parasitic origin | **Osteomyelitis in the oral cavity**

Osteomyelitis and regional soft-tissue lesions from electric cord burns (histopathologically confirmed).

A Lesion on the right lower lip with a soft-tissue defect due to a burn as a result of biting an electric cord.

B Signs of infection of the soft tissue of the lower lip.

C Suspected exposure of non-vital bone tissue.

D RmaxP4 (108).

E RmaxM1(109).

F Image of the osteomyelitis in the region of RmaxP4 (108) and RmaxM1 (109).

G From right to left: RmandP4 (408) and RmandM1 (409).

H Close-up of the osteomyelitis in the region of RmandP4 (408) and RmandM1 (409).

I Close-up of the osteomyelitic portion of bone with RmandP4 (408) and RmandM1 (409) after its removal from the oral cavity.

Key diagnostic/treatment points
Just like in dogs, these lesions are frequent in young cats that have bitten an electric cord, and include soft-tissue injuries, osteomyelitis, and necrosis of the bone tissue. These lesions and infected tissues often cause different degrees of halitosis with signs of oral pain. Their diagnosis and treatment is based on the histopathological confirmation of the process and elimination of the affected tissues, combined with a specific antibiotic treatment.

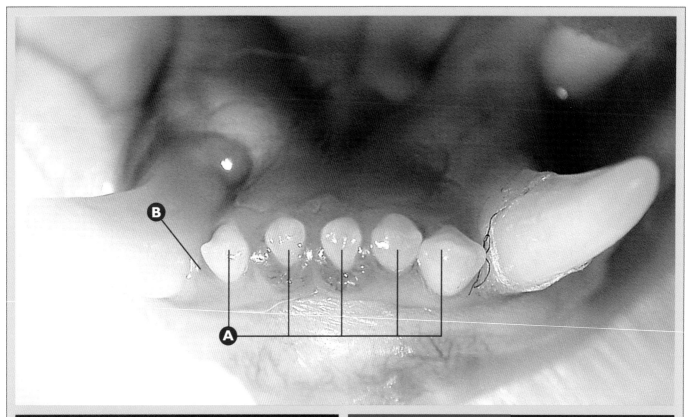

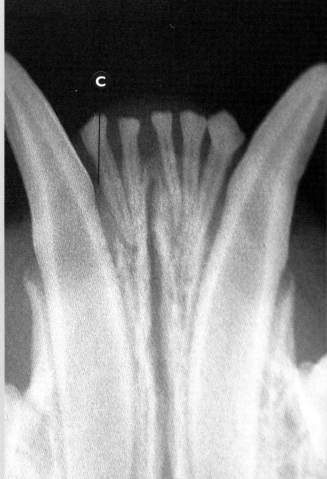

Abnormal dental development and eruption | **Dental agenesis**

Suspected dental agenesis of RmandI3 (403) in a six-month-old patient.

(A) From right to left: LmandI1 (303), LmandI2 (302), LmandI1 (301), RmandI1 (401), RmandI2 (402).

(B) Suspected dental agenesis of RmandI3 (403).

(C) Dental X-ray: radiological signs compatible with agenesis of RmandI1 (403).

Key diagnostic/treatment points

In those young animals that present with a dental absence at the final period of eruption of the permanent teeth, the most probable diagnosis is dental agenesis. However, we cannot rule out a traumatic origin of the absence. Dental X-rays are indispensable to confirm our suspicions.

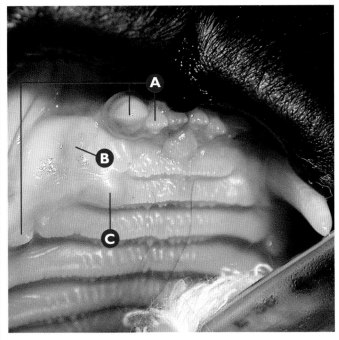

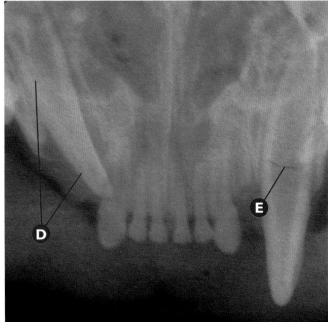

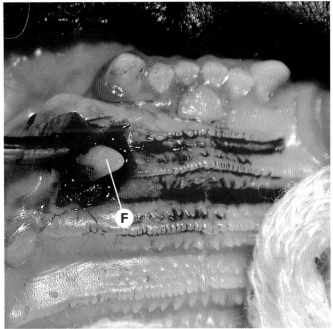

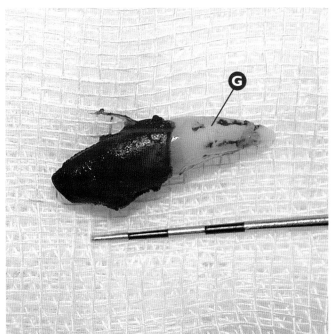

Abnormal dental development and eruption | **Impacted teeth**

Complete impaction of RmaxC (104).

Ⓐ From right to left: RmaxI2 (102), RmaxI3 (103), RmaxP2 (106).

Ⓑ Absence of RmaxC (104).

Ⓒ Area of thickening of the palatal mucosa, leading to suspicions of the presence of a tooth.

Ⓓ Dental X-ray: signs compatible with the presence of RmaxC (104), with complete impaction.

Ⓔ Dental X-ray: artefact.

Ⓕ Close-up of RmaxC (104) during its extraction.

Ⓖ Close-up of RmaxC (104) after its extraction.

Key diagnostic/treatment points
In those clinical cases where a tooth is absent but it can be detected on X-rays, we will likely be faced with a dental impaction. In this clinical case, it is likely that an abnormality in the eruption (rotation and/or deviation) has contributed to the process. The impacted tooth should be closely monitored to avoid regional complications. Non-conservative treatment for the prevention of dental diseases resulting from a dental impaction is extraction.

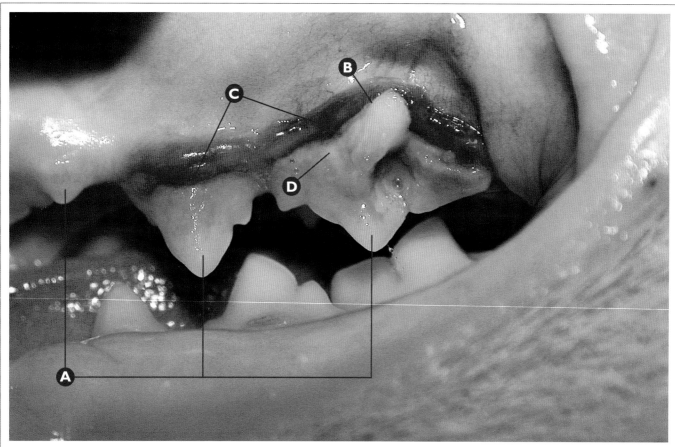

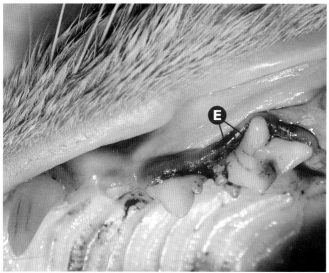

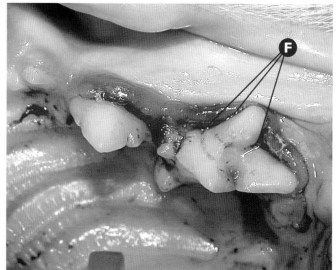

Abnormal dental development and eruption | **Gemination**

Gemination of LmaxP4 (208).

Ⓐ From right to left: LmaxP4 (208), LmaxP3 (207), LmaxP2 (206).

Ⓑ Suspected gemination of LmaxP4 (208).

Ⓒ Gingival index 3 in LmaxP4 (208) and LmaxP3 (207).

Ⓓ Plaque index 3 on LmaxP4 (208).

Ⓔ Gemination of LmaxP4 (208), attempts to form a cusp in the apical area of the vestibular sulcus of the crown of LmaxP4 (208). Image after elimination of the dental plaque and calculus on the tooth surface.

Ⓕ Image of the gemination of LmaxP4 (208).

Key diagnostic/treatment points

Gemination is the attempt to form two teeth from one single dental germ. Gemination in cats is extremely uncommon. Dental X-rays are indicated to assess the root morphology and stage of periodontal disease in this clinical case.

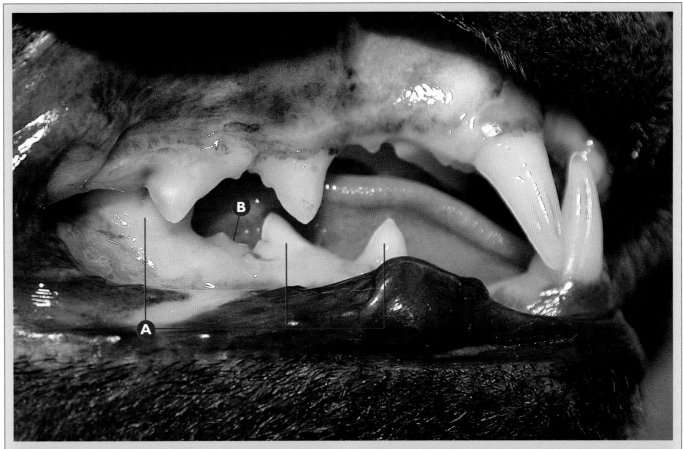

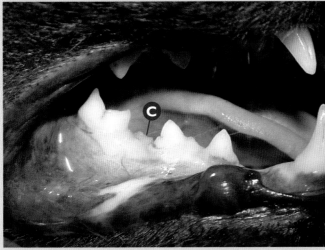

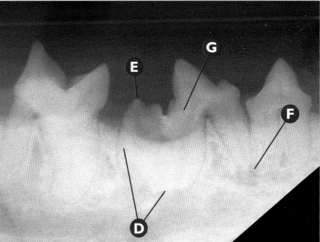

Abnormal dental development and eruption | **Gemination**

Suspected gemination of RmandP4 (408), with a possible fracture.

A From right to left: RmandP3 (407), RmandP4 (408), RmandM1 (409).

B Suspected foreign body distal to RmandP4 (408).

C Image of suspected dental/bone tissue distal to RmandP4 (408).

D Dental X-ray: radiological signs compatible with gemination of RmandP4 (408).

E Dental X-ray: radiological signs compatible with dental tissue (suspicions of a fractured second crown).

F Dental X-ray: radiological signs compatible with periapical disease in the mesial root of RmandP4 (408).

G Dental X-ray: artefact.

Key diagnostic/treatment points

In this clinical case, a gemination of RmandP4 (408) is suspected; this attempt to form two teeth from one single dental germ forms one mesial root and two fused distal roots, with the appearance of one wide distal root. The probable fracture of a second weak distal crown makes it difficult to establish a correct diagnosis. The definitive diagnosis will be reached by histological study of the tooth after extraction, for purely academic purposes.

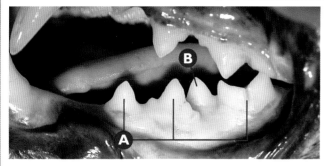

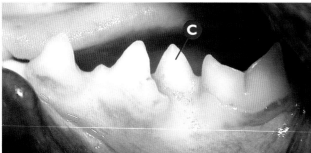

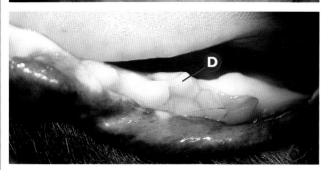

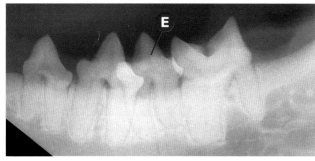

Abnormal dental development and eruption	Hyperdontia (supernumerary teeth)

Presence of a supernumerary tooth, LmandP4' (S308).

Ⓐ From right to left: RmandM1 (309), RmandP4 (308), RmandP3 (307).

Ⓑ LmandP4' (S308); vestibular view.

Ⓒ Close-up of LmandP4' (S308); vestibular view.

Ⓓ Close-up of LmandP4' (S308); occlusal view.

Ⓔ Dental X-ray: radiological signs compatible with LmandP4' (S308).

Key diagnostic/treatment points
A supernumerary tooth is the duplicate of a permanent tooth; in this clinical case it has erupted, causing dental crowding and displacement of the permanent teeth. The presence of this supernumerary tooth favours the progress of the periodontal disease in this region, which may make its extraction indicated.

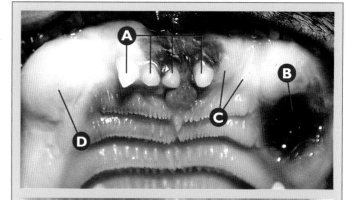

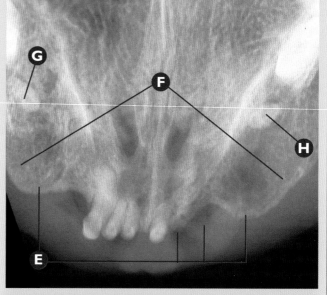

Dental absence

Dental absence of RmaxC (104), LmaxI2 (202), LmaxI3 (203) and LmaxC (204).

Ⓐ From right to left: LmaxI1(201), RmaxI1 (101), RmaxI2 (102), RmaxI3 (103).

Ⓑ Dental absence of LmaxC (204) with open wound, from recent dental loss.

Ⓒ From right to left: dental absence of LmaxI3 (203) and LmaxI2 (202).

Ⓓ Absence of RmaxC (104).

Ⓔ Dental X-ray: from right to left, radiological signs compatible with dental absence of LmaxC (204), LmaxI3 (203), LmaxI2 (202) and RmaxC (104).

Ⓕ Dental X-ray: radiological signs compatible with expansion of the vestibular bone, compatible with advanced stages of periodontal disease.

Ⓖ Dental X-ray: radiological signs compatible with RmaxP2 (106).

Ⓗ Dental X-ray: radiological signs compatible with LmaxP2 (206).

Key diagnostic/treatment points
Dental absence is the visual non-existence of a tooth, with very diverse aetiologies, which can be congenital or acquired. In this case, the absence of RmaxC (104) and LmaxC (204) is most likely due to an advanced stage of periodontal disease, based on the clinical appearance and more particularly on the radiological signs of bone expansion. Another likely differential diagnosis is tooth resorption. In any case, dental X-rays are highly recommended for a tentative or definitive diagnosis of the process.

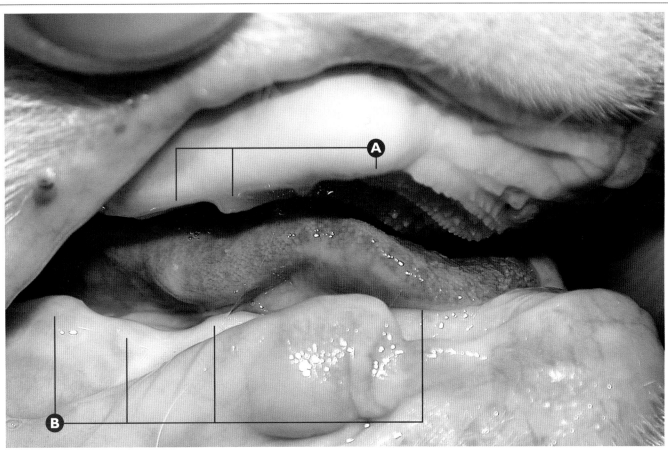

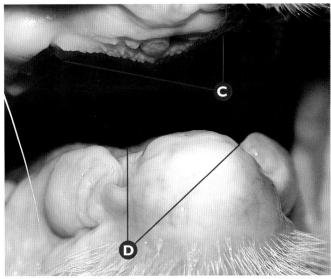

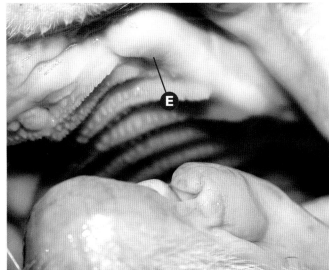

Dental absence

Complete absence of all of the teeth in the oral cavity.

(A) From right to left: absence of RmaxC (104), RmaxP2 (106), RmaxP3 (107).

(B) From right to left: absence of RmandC (404), RmandP3 (407), RmandP4(408), RmandM1(409).

(C) Absence of all the upper incisor teeth.

(D) Absence of all the lower incisor teeth.

(E) Absence of LmaxC (204).

Key diagnostic/treatment points

Dental absence is the visual non-existence of a tooth; in some cases all the teeth may be absent. In most cases, the absence is due to losing teeth as a result of severe periodontal disease (elderly patients); in others animals, the teeth have previously been extracted for different causes (periodontal disease, tooth resorption, feline gingivostomatitis, etc.). These animals can lead completely normal lives and eat without any difficulties. Occasionally, the only defect is aesthetic, with partial exposure of the tongue outside the oral cavity when the animal is at rest.

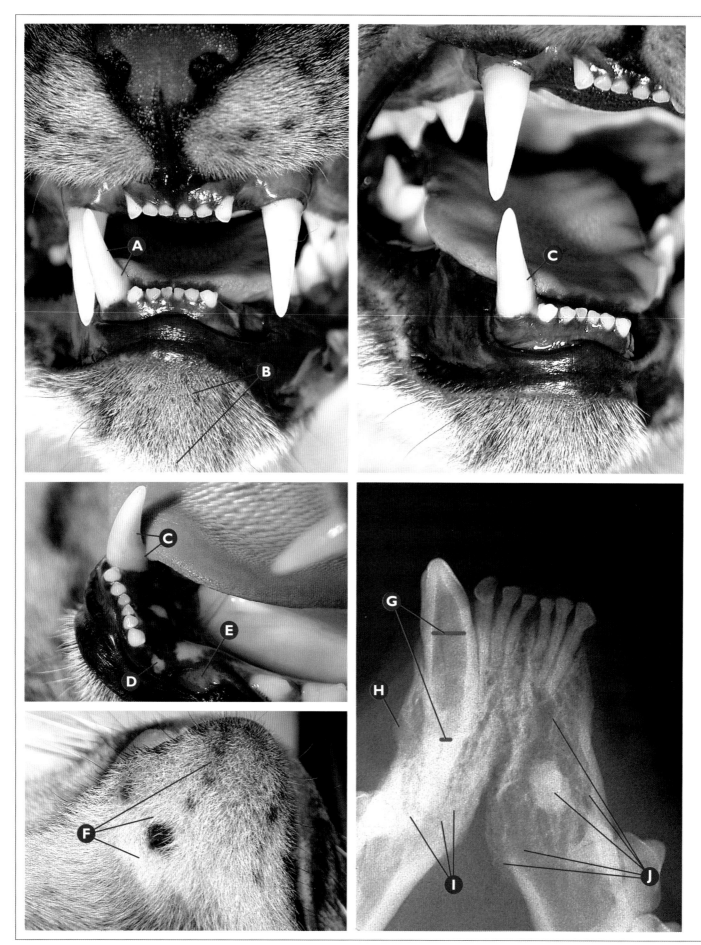

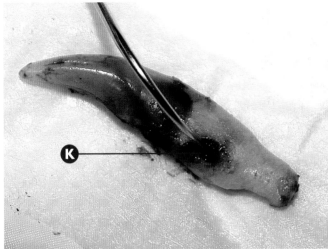

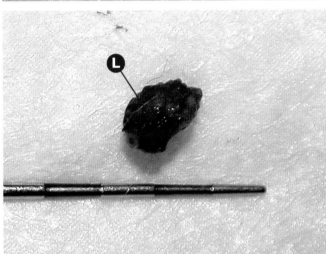

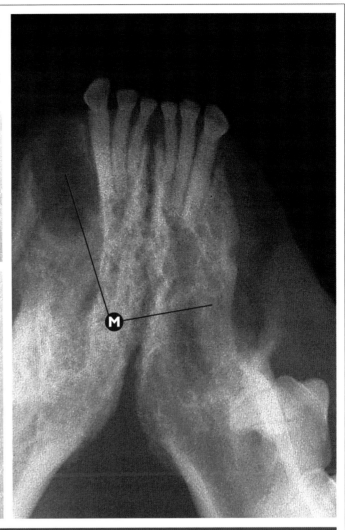

Dental discolouration

Discolouration of the apical and middle third of the crown of RmandC (404) due to endodontic disease; dark brown colouration.

Ⓐ Dark brown discolouration of the crown of RmandC (404).

Ⓑ Mandibular abscess on the chin and symphyseal area.

Ⓒ Image of the discolouration of the crown of RmandC (404).

Ⓓ Absence of LmandC (304).

Ⓔ Mandibular abscess in the vestibular region of LmandC (304) (absent).

Ⓕ Close-up of the mandibular abscess in the chin and symphyseal area, with a fistulous tract to the exterior.

Ⓖ Dental X-ray: radiological signs compatible with endodontic disease (pulp necrosis) in RmandC (404).

Ⓗ Dental X-ray: radiological signs compatible with osteolysis in the vestibular bone of RmandC (404).

Ⓘ Dental X-ray: radiological signs compatible with a periapical granuloma at RmandC (404).

Ⓙ Dental X-ray: radiological signs compatible with a retained root of LmandC (304), with signs of osteolysis in this region.

Ⓚ Close-up of RmandC (404) with perforation in the root and communication with the pulp chamber, after its extraction.

Ⓛ Close-up of the retained root of LmandC (304), after its extraction.

Ⓜ Dental X-ray: radiological signs compatible with the absence of RmandC (404) and LmandC (304); after surgical treatment.

Key diagnostic/treatment points
Endodontic disease (pulp necrosis) is the most probable aetiology of this dental discolouration. It has caused a periapical granuloma and regional dental abscess. The abscess observed in the vestibular region of LmandC (304) is likely due to the retained root of this tooth. Dental X-rays must be performed in cases of dental discolouration to determine its origin. In this clinical case, non-conservative treatment includes the extraction of both RmandC (404) and the retained root of LmandC (304).

Common errors
Underestimating the importance of dental discolouration, even if the tooth seems intact. Advanced periodontal disease, as well as pulp necrosis, may cause discolouration without apparently affecting the integrity of the crown.

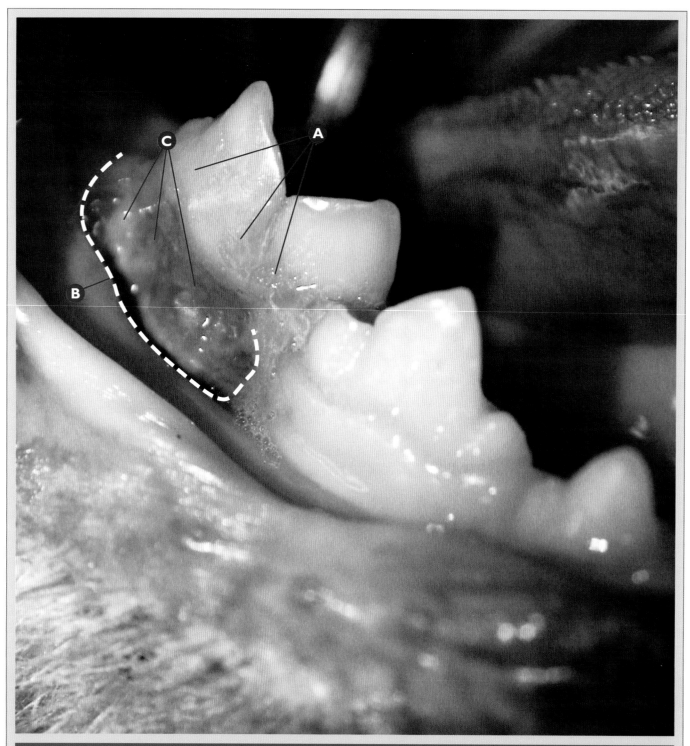

Dental discolouration

Discolouration of the apical and middle third of the crown of RmandM1 (409); dark purple colouration.

Ⓐ Dark purple discolouration in the apical third of the crown of RmandM1 (409).

Ⓑ Severe gingival recession and severe loss of the bone surrounding RmandM1 (409).

Ⓒ Suspected stage 4 periodontal disease in RmandM1 (409).

Key diagnostic/treatment points

In this case, dental discolouration is most likely due to advanced periodontal disease. Dental discolouration may be caused by irreversible pulpitis or pulp necrosis. Adequate treatment in this clinical case will be dental extraction once the stage 4 periodontal disease is confirmed.

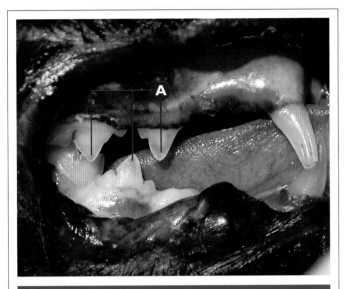

Dental discolouration

Discolouration with increase in the transparency of the tooth, due to advanced age.

A From right to left: increased dental transparency (enamel and dentin) in RmaxP3 (107), RmandP4 (408) and RmaxP4 (108).

Key diagnostic/treatment points
In very old animals, an increase in tooth transparency is often detected, with the most accepted aetiology being the progressive demineralisation of the teeth with age.

| Dental fracture | Enamel fracture |

Enamel fracture of the cusp of LmaxC (204).

A Enamel fracture of the cusp of LmaxC (204).

B Ulcer in the distovestibular mucosa of LmandC (304), suspected ulcer from contact/occlusion of LmaxC (204).

C Close-up of the enamel fracture of the cusp of LmaxC (204).

D Plaque index 3 on LmaxC (204).

E Bacterial plaque from scraping the periodontal probe over the palatal surface of LmaxC (204).

Key diagnostic/treatment points
Single enamel fractures in cats are uncommon; tooth resorption is occasionally misdiagnosed for enamel fractures. The detection of a fracture only of the cusp of the tooth leads us to suspect an enamel fracture. The ulcer in the mucosa of the lower lip is likely caused by the trauma of the cutting edge of the fractured enamel as well as the constant contact with the palatal surface of LmaxC (204); it is probably infected due to contact with the accumulation of bacterial plaque on the palatal surface of LmaxC (204). These enamel fractures have no clinical significance other than the occasions on which the cutting edges may cause lesions to soft tissues.

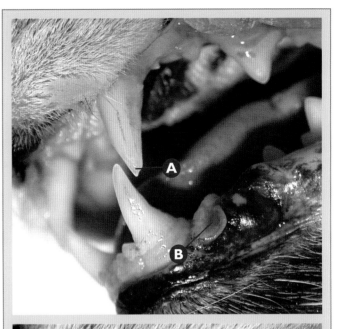
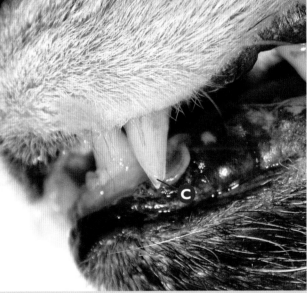
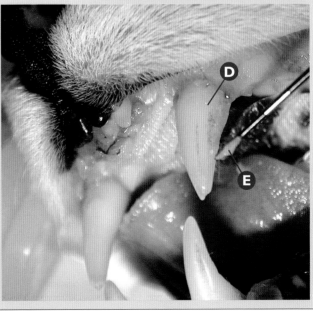

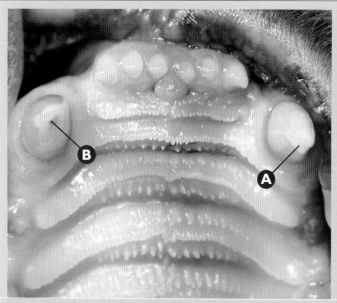
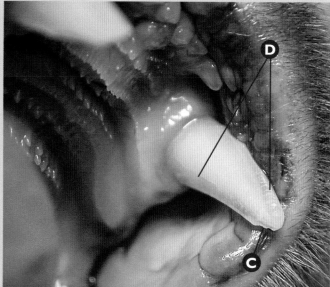

Dental fracture | Enamel fracture

Enamel fracture of the cusp of LmaxC (204).

Ⓐ Suspected enamel fracture of the cusp of LmaxC (204).

Ⓑ Suspicions of a complicated crown fracture of RmaxC (104).

Ⓒ Close-up of the enamel fracture on the cusp of LmaxC (204).

Ⓓ Enamel infraction in LmaxC (204).

Key diagnostic/treatment points

These very small-sized enamel fractures have no clinical significance and do not require dental treatment (after radiological confirmation of the process). Occasionally, the dental edges of the enamel caused by the fracture may cause mild lesions to the surrounding soft tissues. These irregularities in the enamel may be removed using a turbine and fine diamond burs.

Dental fracture | Uncomplicated crown fracture

Uncomplicated crown fracture of LmaxC (204).

Ⓐ Uncomplicated crown fracture of LmaxC (204).

Ⓑ Enamel (fractured).

Ⓒ Dentin (fractured).

Key diagnostic/treatment points

Uncomplicated fractures of the coronal third of the crown of the canine teeth are uncommon in cats. Trauma to this region, the most frequent cause of this condition in these teeth, tends to expose the pulp. When only 1–2 mm of the cusp fractures away, the pulp chamber will sometimes not be exposed and an uncomplicated crown fracture will occur, as in this clinical case.

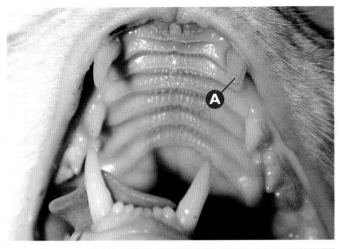

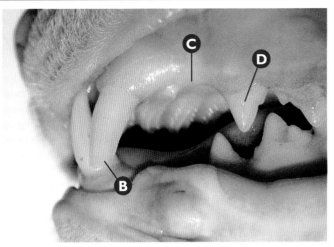

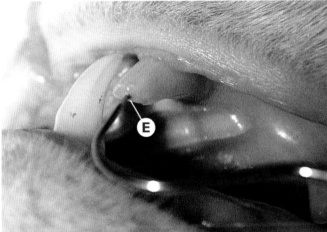

Dental fracture | Complicated crown fracture

Relatively recent complicated crown fracture of LmaxC (204).

Ⓐ Suspicions of a complicated crown fracture of LmaxC (204).

Ⓑ Suspicions of a complicated crown fracture of LmaxC (204); vestibular view.

Ⓒ Absence of LmaxP2 (206).

Ⓓ Calculus index 1 on LmaxP3 (207).

Ⓔ Confirmation of the complicated crown fracture of LmaxC (204), using a dental explorer.

Ⓕ Dental X-ray: radiological signs compatible with pulp chambers with similar diameters in RmaxC (104) and LmaxC (204).

Ⓖ Dental X-ray: radiological signs compatible with complicated crown fracture of LmaxC (204).

Ⓗ Dental X-ray: radiological signs compatible with mild root resorption in the apical region of LmaxC (204). Stage 2 tooth resorption.

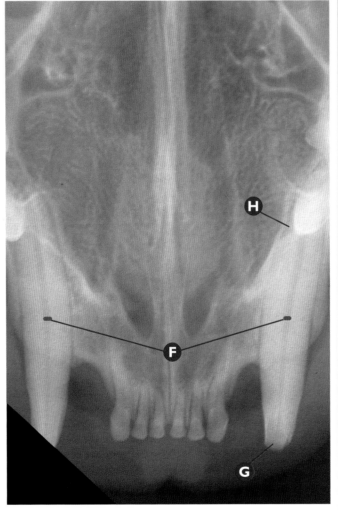

Key diagnostic/treatment points
In complicated crown fractures in cats, the loss of dental tissue may be minimal, and many times they go unnoticed. On this occasion, since the diameters of the pulp chambers of both upper canine teeth are similar (radiologically), we can consider that the fracture is relatively recent. However, the apical lesion of LmaxC (204) may be compatible with a periapical disease caused by this type of fracture. A lateral occlusal dental X-ray should be performed to assess the true extent of the root resorption of LmaxC (204) as well as the possibility that the lesion may be caused by tooth resorption.

Common errors
If an adequate definitive oral examination is not performed (using a dental explorer and with the animal sedated), many of the dental fractures that present with a slight loss of dental tissue will be underdiagnosed, and providing appropriate treatment will be impossible.

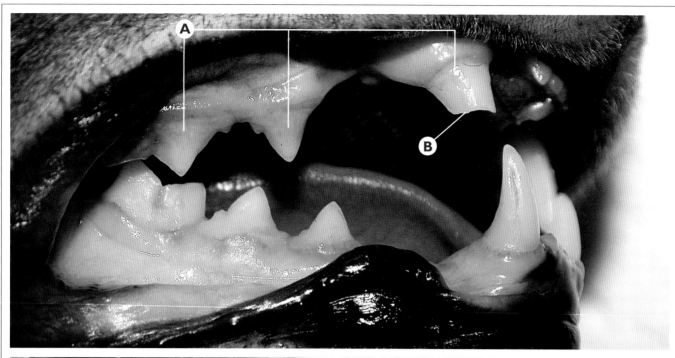

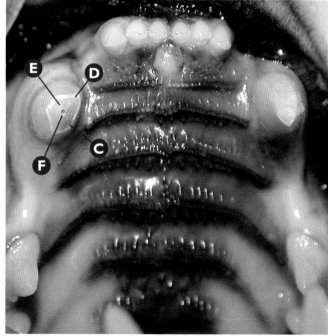

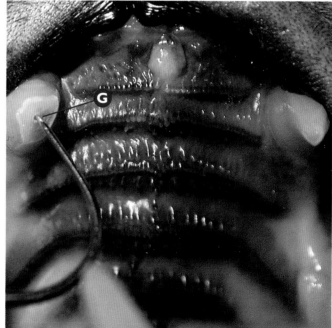

Dental fracture | **Complicated crown fracture**

Complicated crown fracture of RmaxC (104).

Ⓐ From right to left: RmaxC (104), RmaxP3 (107) and RmaxP4 (108).

Ⓑ Suspicions of a complicated crown fracture of RmaxC (104); right vestibular view.

Ⓒ Complicated crown fracture of RmaxC (104); coronal view.

Ⓓ Fractured enamel.

Ⓔ Fractured dentin.

Ⓕ Pulp cavity of RmaxC (104) exposed.

Ⓖ Image of the complicated crown fracture of RmaxC (104), using a dental explorer; coronal view.

Key diagnostic/treatment points

Complicated crown fractures of the canine teeth are relatively common in cats. In fractures where there is no severe loss of dental tissue, a conservative treatment option can be suggested, such as pulpectomy (after assessment using dental X-rays). If the owner declines the conservative treatment or it is not viable, dental extraction will be the adequate treatment.

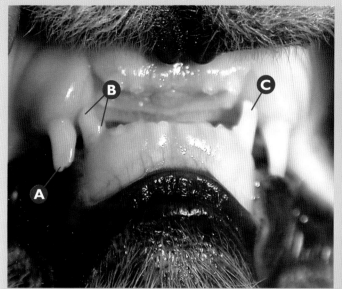

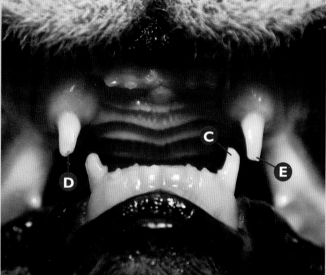

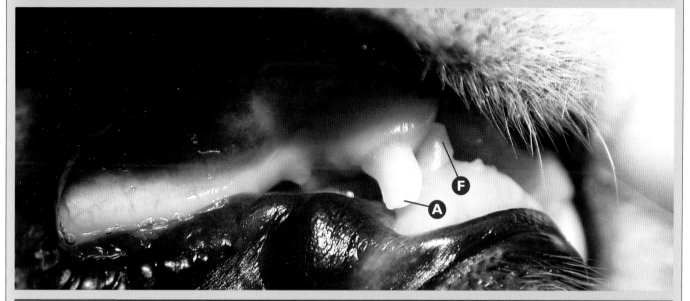

Dental fracture | **Complicated crown fracture**

Complicated crown fracture in deciduous canine teeth: RmaxC (504), LmaxC (604), LmandC (704) and RmandC (804) in a 4-month-old cat; iatrogenic aetiology.

Ⓐ Complicated crown fracture of deciduous RmaxC (504).

Ⓑ Suspected complicated crown fracture of deciduous RmandC (804), with visible dental discolouration.

Ⓒ Suspected complicated crown fracture of deciduous LmandC (704).

Ⓓ Image of the complicated crown fracture of deciduous RmaxC (504); with pulp necrosis.

Ⓔ Suspicions of a complicated crown fracture of LmaxC (604).

Ⓕ Dental discolouration in deciduous RmandC (804).

Key diagnostic/treatment points
From time to time, especially in show animals of a very young age, we can observe complicated crown fractures of the deciduous canine teeth caused by their owners in a iatrogenic manner, supposedly to correct, modify, or avoid dental malocclusions. These fractures are produced by cutting the cusps of the deciduous canine teeth with scissors or pliers, sometimes without anaesthesia. This concept is as incorrect as it is inhumane for our patients, and involves deliberately causing a complicated crown fracture, with its respective unjustified pain when exposing the live pulp. When causing these dental fractures, not only are the malocclusions not corrected, but the very consequences of the complicated fractures themselves are caused in a deciduous tooth (pulp necrosis and even involvement of the dental germ of the corresponding permanent tooth). The discolouration detected in these teeth is due to the necrosis of their pulp.

Common errors
Not reeducating the client by explaining the erroneous nature of these actions and concepts, and not informing about the horrible consequences of these iatrogenic complicated fractures.

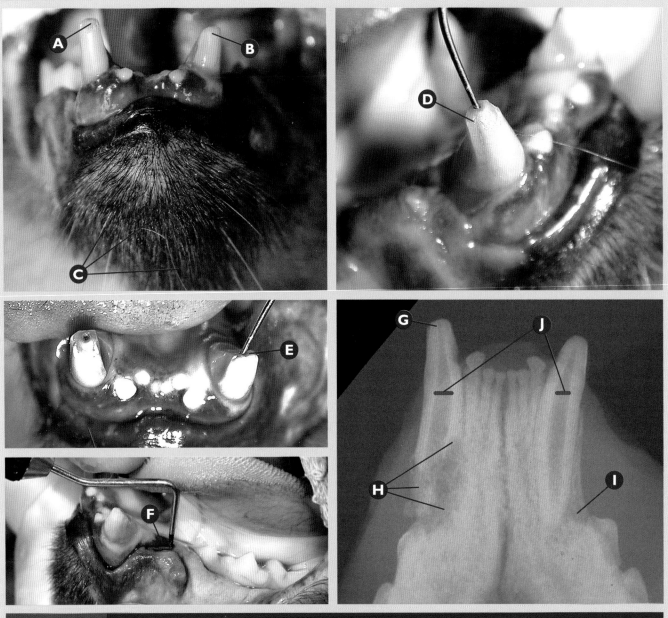

Dental fracture | Complicated crown fracture

Complicated crown fracture of LmandC (304) and RmandC (404), which has caused an abscess in the mandibular symphyseal region in an adult cat.

Ⓐ Suspicions of a complicated crown fracture of RmandC (404).

Ⓑ Suspicions of a complicated crown fracture of LmandC (304).

Ⓒ Severe mandibular abscess in the region of the mandibular symphysis.

Ⓓ Confirmation of the complicated crown fracture of RmandC (404), using a dental explorer.

Ⓔ Confirmation of the complicated crown fracture of LmandC (304), using a dental explorer.

Ⓕ Fistulous tract in the mucosa distal to LmandC (304), with production of sero-sanguinolent fluid, and a depth of 10 mm measured with a periodontal probe.

Ⓖ Dental X-ray: radiological signs compatible with a complicated crown fracture of RmandC (404).

Ⓗ Dental X-ray: radiological signs compatible with periapical osteolysis and severe root resorption (stage 4c tooth resorption) of RmandC (404).

Ⓘ Dental X-ray: radiological signs compatible with moderate/severe osteolysis in the periapical area of LmandC (304).

Ⓙ Dental X-ray: radiological signs compatible with wider pulp cavities than those that correspond with the animal's adult age.

Key diagnostic/treatment points
Complicated crown fractures in the canine teeth must be treated as soon as they are detected, with conservative or non-conservative treatment. Although no signs of endodontic disease are visible at first, the pulp necrosis will progress and cause periapical disease which may even lead to a dental abscess, such as in this clinical case. The non-conservative treatment in this clinical case would be the extraction of both canine teeth.

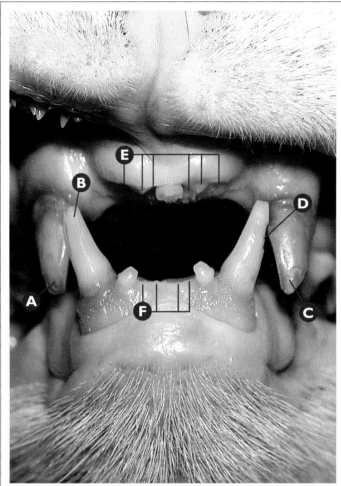

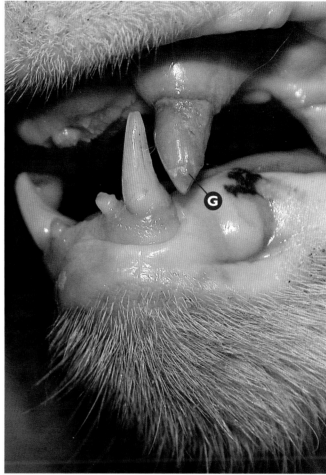

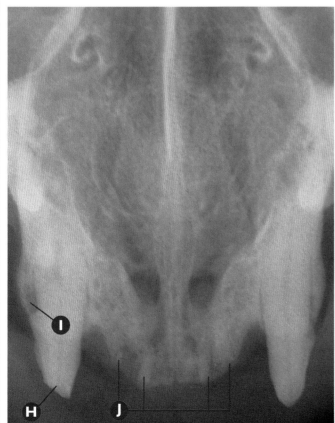

Complicated crown fracture of RmaxC (104).

Ⓐ Complicated crown fracture of RmaxC (104); rostral view.

Ⓑ Suspicions of an uncomplicated crown fracture of RmandC (404).

Ⓒ Suspicions of a complicated crown fracture of LmaxC (204).

Ⓓ Enamel fracture of LmandC (304).

Ⓔ Absence of all the upper incisor teeth.

Ⓕ From right to left: absence of LmandI2 (302), LmandI1 (301), RmandI1 (401) and RmandI2 (402).

Ⓖ Suspicions of a complicated crown fracture of LmaxC (204).

Ⓗ Dental X-ray: radiological signs compatible with a complicated crown fracture of RmaxC (104).

Ⓘ Dental X-ray: radiological signs compatible with expansion of the vestibular bone in RmaxC (104).

Ⓙ Dental X-ray: radiological signs compatible with stage 5 tooth resorption in the maxillary incisor teeth.

Key diagnostic/treatment points

The macroscopic aspect of the teeth and dental X-rays will not always be determinant to establish if the fracture is complicated or not. We can sometimes see the opening to the pulp cavity with the naked eye (complicated fracture) or on the X-rays. On other occasions, however, the use of a dental explorer will be essential for a correct dental examination.

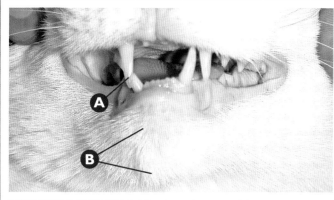

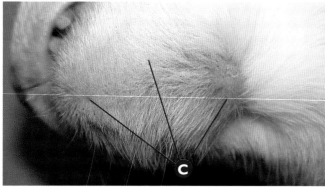

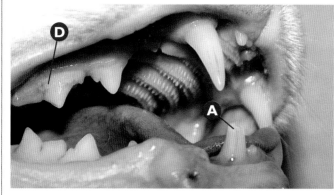

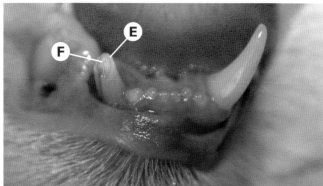

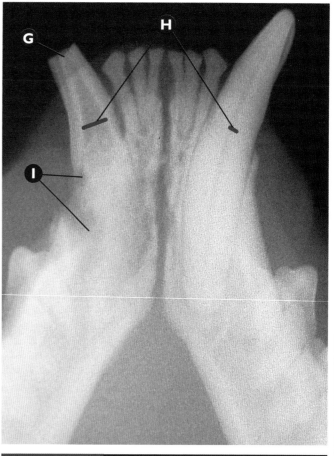

Dental fracture | **Complicated crown fracture**

Complicated crown fracture of RmandC (404), causing a mandibular abscess in the symphyseal region in an adult cat.

Ⓐ Suspicions of a complicated crown fracture of RmandC (404).

Ⓑ Severe mandibular abscess in the region of the mandibular symphysis.

Ⓒ Image of the mandibular abscess in the chin and mandibular symphysis area.

Ⓓ Plaque index 3 on RmaxP4 (108).

Ⓔ Confirmation of a complicated crown fracture of RmandC (404).

Ⓕ Exposure of the pulp cavity in RmandC (404), caused by a complicated fracture.

Ⓖ Dental X-ray: radiological signs compatible with a complicated crown fracture of RmandC (404).

Ⓗ Dental X-ray: radiological signs compatible with a wide pulp cavity compared with that of the left mandibular canine tooth, which would indicate a previous fracture.

Ⓘ Dental X-ray: radiological signs compatible with osteolysis and severe resorption of the root of RmandC (404).

Key diagnostic/treatment points
This clinical case shows us once again that when small dental fractures with presence of pulp exposure are detected, they should be treated as soon as possible after performing a dental radiological study. The progress to pulp necrosis is more than obvious and has led to a dental abscess, even though years have passed since the complicated fracture occurred. RmandC (404) must be extracted.

Common errors
Not giving enough importance to the diagnosis and treatment of dental fractures, especially in those cases of polytraumatised animals. In animals that have received trauma to the oral cavity (run over by a vehicle, falls from great heights...), we must perform an in-depth study of the oral cavity to assess any changes to the hard and soft tissues, together with a complete dental examination.

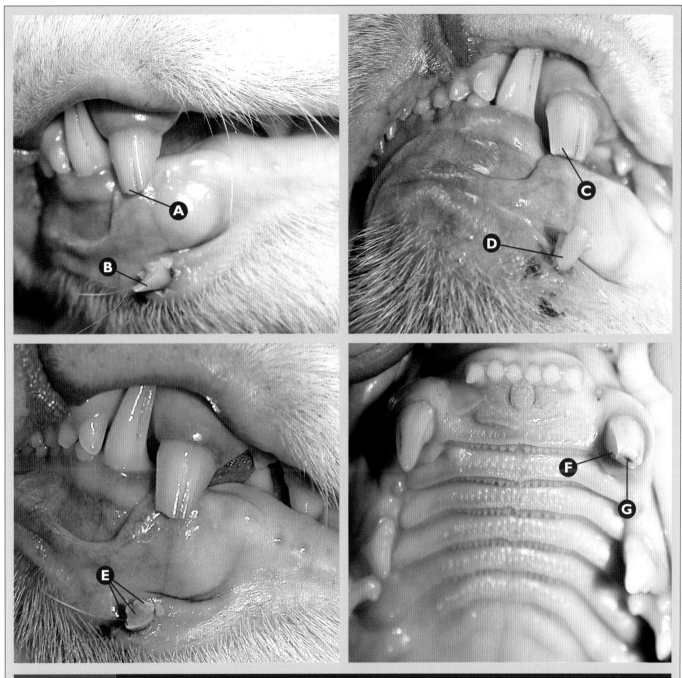

Dental fracture | **Complicated crown fracture**

Very recent complicated crown fracture of LmaxC (204).

Ⓐ Suspicions of a complicated crown fracture of LmaxC (204); vestibular view.

Ⓑ Cusp of LmaxC (204), stabbed into the mucosa of the lower left lip.

Ⓒ Complicated crown fracture of LmaxC (204).

Ⓓ Image of the cusp of LmaxC (204), stabbed into the mucosa of the lower left lip.

Ⓔ Image of the affected dental structures in the dental fracture.

Ⓕ Confirmation of a complicated crown fracture of LmaxC (204).

Ⓖ Vital dental pulp of LmaxC (204).

Key diagnostic/treatment points
Very occasionally, we can detect signs that the dental fractures are extremely recent. This patient suffered a moderate injury 30 minutes before the examination. The fact that the fractured cusp of LmaxC (204) has remained impacted into the lower lip confirms this. In a short period of time, this soft tissue will present with moderate inflammation, causing the dehiscence of the cusp. The recommended treatment in this case of very recent complicated crown fracture can be conservative (partial coronal pulpectomy), or non-conservative (extraction). The absence of collateral damage must be confirmed by dental X-rays.

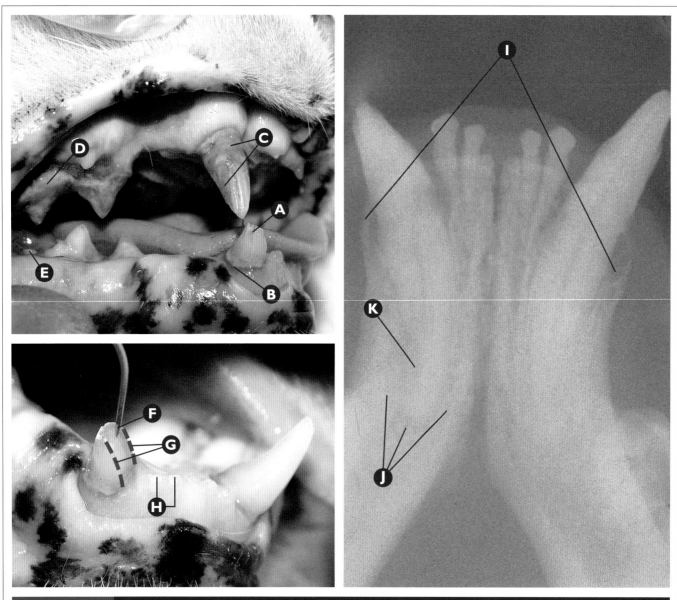

Dental fracture   Complicated crown-root fracture

Complicated crown-root fracture of RmandC (404).

Ⓐ Suspicions of a complicated crown-root fracture of RmandC (404).

Ⓑ Gingival index 1 in RmandC (404).

Ⓒ Calculus index 3 on RmaxC (104).

Ⓓ Plaque index 4 on RmaxP4 (108).

Ⓔ Suspected stage 4b tooth resorption in RmandM1 (409).

Ⓕ Confirmation of the complicated crown-root fracture of RmandC (404), using a dental explorer.

Ⓖ Close-up of the fracture line towards the subgingival area of RmandC (404).

Ⓗ From right to left: attrition of RmandI2 (402) and RmandI3 (403).

Ⓘ From right to left: dental X-ray: radiological signs compatible with expansion of the vestibular bone of LmandC (304) and RmandC (404), compatible with periodontal disease.

Ⓙ Dental X-ray: radiological signs compatible with severe osteolysis in the periapical region of RmandC (404).

Ⓚ Dental X-ray: radiological signs compatible with severe resorption of the root (stage 3 tooth resorption) of RmandC (404), due to endodontic disease.

Key diagnostic/treatment points

In complicated crown-root fractures, there is exposure of the pulp chamber and the fracture extends below the cementoenamel junction. If we do not treat this problem appropriately and in a timely manner, this exposure of the pulp will cause pulp necrosis (as has already occurred in this clinical case). A narrow pulp chamber with a diameter similar to its lower counterpart indicates that the fracture has taken place at an adult age. However, this fracture is not very recent as there is endodontic disease that can be detected radiologically, with signs that are compatible with root resorption and periapical osteolysis. In this case, the most appropriate treatment is the extraction of the tooth, given that conservative endodontic treatment (pulpectomy) would not be viable due to the severe loss of dental tissue in the root.

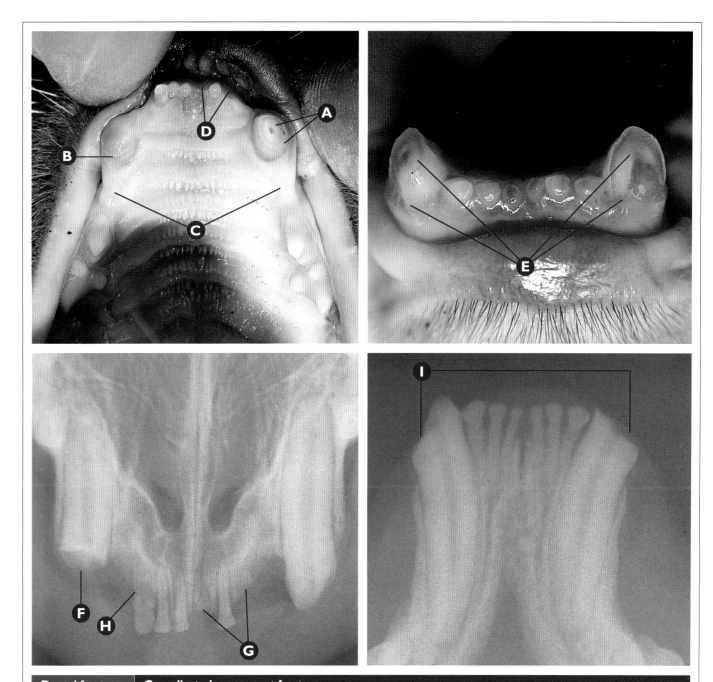

Dental fracture | **Complicated crown-root fracture**

Complicated crown-root fracture of RmaxC (104), LmandC (304) and RmandC (404).

A Complicated crown fracture of LmaxC (204), with exposure of pulp that is still vital.

B Complicated crown-root fracture of RmaxC (104).

C Absence of RmaxP2 (106) and LmaxP2 (206).

D From right to left: absence of LmaxI3 (203) and LmaxI1 (201).

E From right to left: complicated crown-root fracture of LmandC (304) and RmandC (404).

F Dental X-ray: radiological signs compatible with a complicated crown-root fracture of RmaxC (101).

G Dental X-ray: radiological signs compatible with stage 4b tooth resorption of LmaxI1 (201) and LmaxI3 (203).

H Dental X-ray: radiological signs compatible with stage 4c tooth resorption of RmaxI3 (103).

I Dental X-ray: (from right to left) radiological signs compatible with a complicated crown fracture of LmandC (304) and RmandC (404).

Key diagnostic/treatment points
Multiple dental fractures of different types are often seen in the same oral cavity. Each of the affected teeth should be classified and treatment should be provided according to each type of dental fracture. Non-conservative treatment of these complicated crown-root fractures is dental extraction.

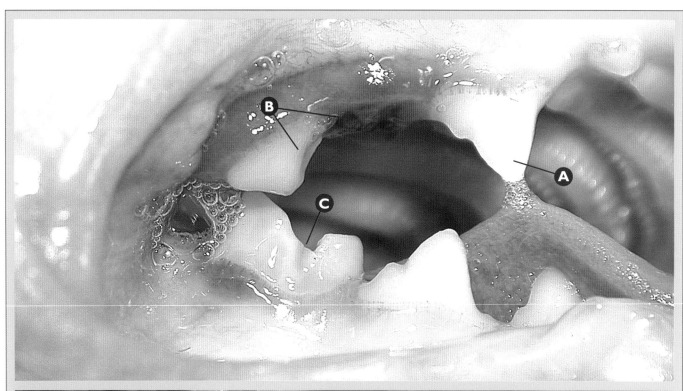

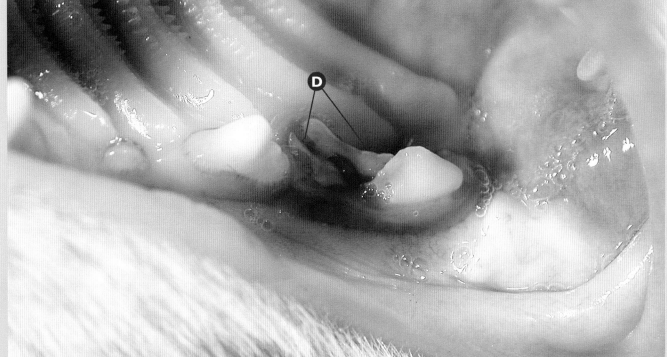

Dental fracture   Complicated crown-root fracture

Complicated crown-root fracture of RmaxP4 (108).

A RmaxP3 (107).

B Complicated crown-root fracture of RmaxP4 (108).

C Suspicions of an uncomplicated crown fracture of RmandM1 (409).

D Close-up of a complicated crown-root fracture of RmaxP4 (108).

Key diagnostic/treatment points
This type of fracture often has a traumatic aetiology. The uncomplicated crown fracture of RmandM1 (409), a regional tooth, further supports our suspicions as to the cause of the fracture. Treatment of this type of complicated crown-root fractures is dental extraction, after performing a regional dental radiological study.

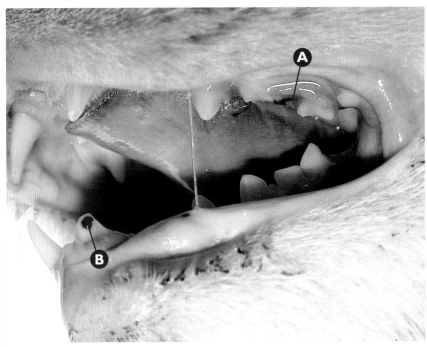

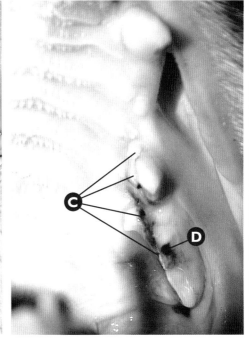

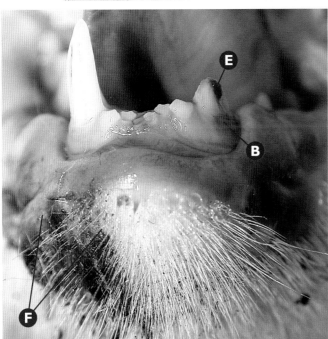

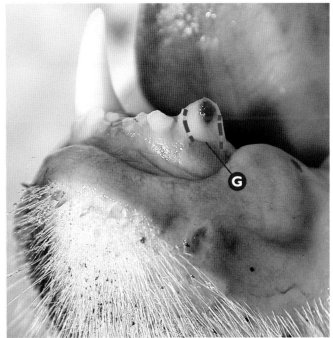

Dental fracture   **Complicated crown-root fracture**

Complicated crown-root fracture of LmaxP3 (207), LmaxP4 (208) and LmandC (304); trauma caused by a fall from great heights.

Ⓐ Suspicions of a complicated crown-root fracture of LmaxP4 (208).

Ⓑ Suspicions of a complicated crown-root fracture of LmandC (304).

Ⓒ Confirmation of the complicated crown-root fracture of LmaxP3 (207) and LmaxP4 (208).

Ⓓ Exposed vital pulp of LmaxP4 (208).

Ⓔ Exposed vital pulp of LmandC (304).

Ⓕ Severe lesion of the lower lip due to the trauma.

Ⓖ Confirmation of a complicated crown-root fracture of LmandC (304).

Key diagnostic/treatment points

Trauma as a result of a patient falling from great heights may cause dental lesions, primarily dental fractures, along with lesions to soft tissues and bone tissues closely related to the oral cavity. In these recent complicated fractures, we can observe exposed vital pulp and signs of pulp inflammation.

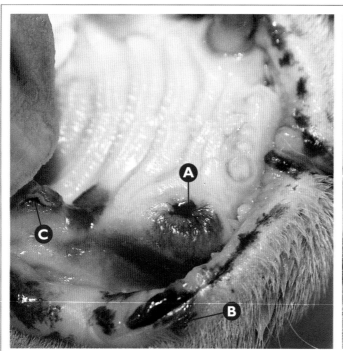

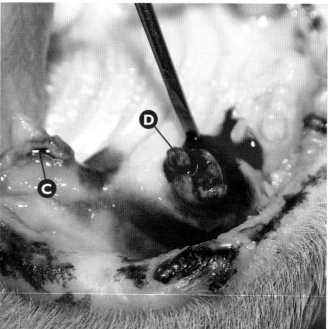

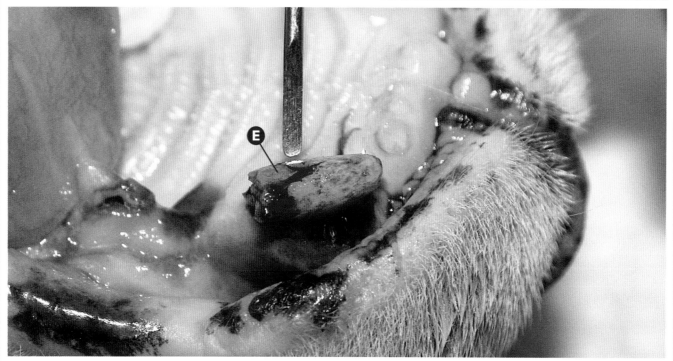

| Dental fracture | Root fracture |

Recent root fracture of LmaxC (204).

Ⓐ Absence of LmaxC (204), with history of trauma and fracture in the last 48 hours.

Ⓑ Lesion in the upper lip in the LmaxC (204) region.

Ⓒ Suspected stage 3 tooth resorption of LmaxP3 (207).

Ⓓ Image of the luxation of the root fragment of LmaxC (204), with a Davis root elevator (Hu-Friedy® ED11).

Ⓔ Root fragment of LmaxC (204).

Key diagnostic/treatment points

When dental trauma is recent, we must ask the patient's owner to keep the fragment of the fractured tooth if possible. This will provide us with valuable information regarding the existence or lack of a retained root. Regional dental X-rays in these cases are mandatory. Treatment of root fractures is based on the extraction of the retained root(s).

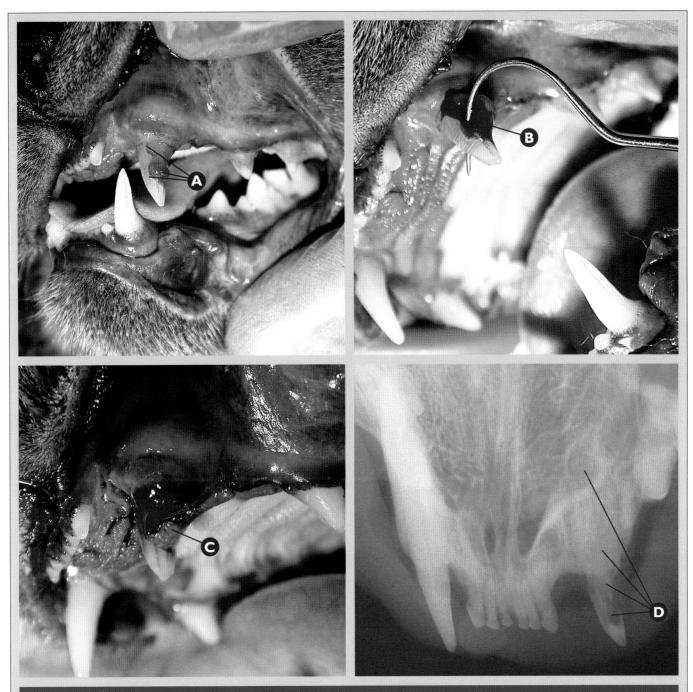

Tooth resorption

Stage 4 tooth resorption of LmaxC (204).

A Suspicions of stage 4 tooth resorption of LmaxC (204), with loss of dental tissue (enamel and dentin).

B Use of a dental explorer to confirm the absence of dental tissue in LmaxC (204).

C Image of the severe enamel and dentin defects in LmaxC (204).

D Dental X-ray: radiological signs compatible with stage 4a tooth resorption of LmaxC (204).

Key diagnostic/treatment points

Tooth resorption is a very common disease in felines in general; it has been more particularly detected and studied in cats. Its aetiology, in spite of the studies conducted, is currently unknown. This disease causes the destruction of dental tissue due to the activation of the osteoclasts in the neck and/or root and/or crown of the tooth. A high degree of dental destruction is observed in advanced cases (stage 5). Dental X-rays are an indispensable diagnostic method to determine the degree of dental involvement.

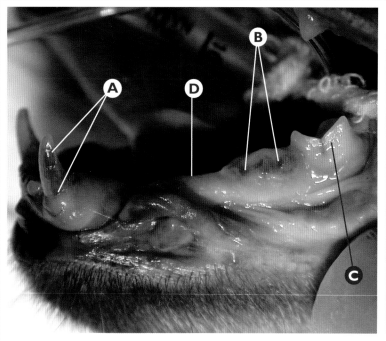

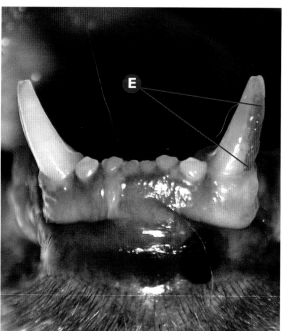

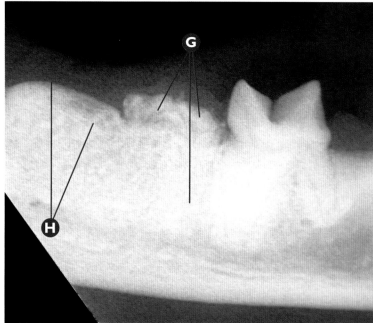

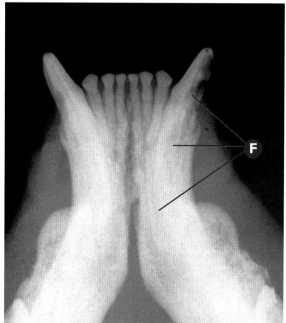

Tooth resorption

Stage 4 feline tooth resorption of LmandC (304) and LmandP4 (308).

Ⓐ Suspicions of stage 4 tooth resorption of LmandC (304).

Ⓑ Suspicions of stage 4 tooth resorption of LmandP4 (308), with severe destruction of the dental structure.

Ⓒ LmandM1 (309).

Ⓓ Absence of LmandP3 (307).

Ⓔ Image of the suspicions of stage 4 tooth resorption of LmandC (304).

Ⓕ Dental X-ray: radiological signs compatible with stage 4a tooth resorption due to severe destruction of the dental structure of LmandC (304).

Ⓖ Dental X-ray: radiological signs compatible with stage 4a tooth resorption of LmandP4 (308).

Ⓗ Dental X-ray: radiological signs compatible with stage 5 tooth resorption of LmandP3 (307).

Key diagnostic/treatment points

In cases of tooth resorption, dental X-rays are an indispensable diagnostic method to determine the exact degree of dental involvement. In this clinical case, the macroscopic aspect of LmandP4 (308) gives us sufficient information to identify the stage of tooth resorption (stage 4). However, a dental radiological assessment is essential to determine the degree of destruction of the dental structure of LmandC (304).

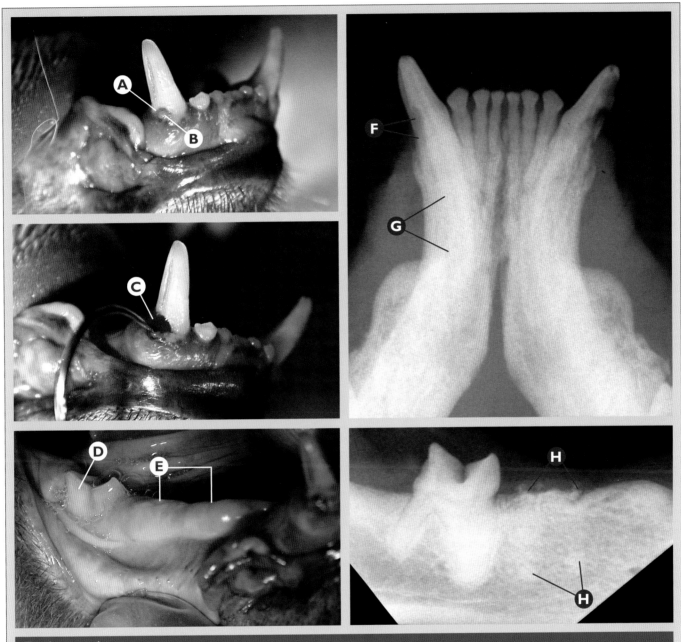

Tooth resorption

Stage 4 tooth resorption of RmandC (404). (Previous case continued).

A Suspicions of stage 2 tooth resorption of RmandC (404).

B Image of gingival hyperplasia in the area of RmandC (404), typical of the initial stages of tooth resorption.

C Image of the suspicions of stage 2 tooth resorption of RmandC (404) with destruction of enamel and dentin, assessed with a dental explorer.

D RmandM1 (409).

E From right to left: absence of RmandP3 (407) and RmandP4 (408).

F Dental X-ray: radiological signs compatible with destruction of the enamel and dentin in RmandC (404), due to tooth resorption.

G Dental X-ray: radiological signs compatible with stage 4 tooth resorption due to severe destruction of the dental structure of RmandC (404).

H Dental X-ray: radiological signs compatible with stage 5 tooth resorption in RmandP4 (408).

Key diagnostic/treatment points
A similar situation is detected on the right mandibular side of the patient from the previous case. The greatest difference lies in the fact that the suspicions of stage 2 tooth resorption of RmandC (404), detected with a dental explorer in the definitive oral examination, are later classified as stage 4 due to the radiological signs of severe destruction in the root of this tooth.

Common errors
Classifying the tooth resorption stage only by oral examination. Dental X-rays are indispensable to detect the true stage of tooth resorption.

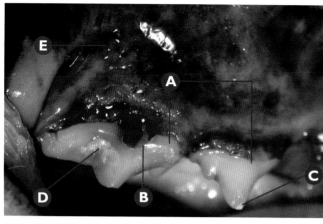

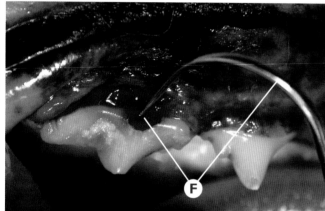

Tooth resorption

Suspicions of stage 3 tooth resorption of RmaxP4 (108).

Ⓐ From right to left: RmaxP3 (107) and RmaxP4 (108).

Ⓑ Suspicions of stage 3 tooth resorption of RmaxP4 (108).

Ⓒ Enamel fracture of RmaxP3 (107).

Ⓓ Calculus index 1 on RmaxP4 (108).

Ⓔ Papilla of the duct of the parotid gland.

Ⓕ Image of the confirmation of the suspicions of stage 3 tooth resorption of RmaxP4 (108) with a dental explorer, with loss of dental tissue (enamel and dentin) and pulp exposure.

Key diagnostic/treatment points
The use of a dental explorer is sometimes indispensable to assess tooth resorption lesions. In this case, it is possible to determine, using the explorer, that dental destruction has reached the pulp chamber. The most appropriate non-conservative treatment is dental extraction, after performing a regional dental radiological study.

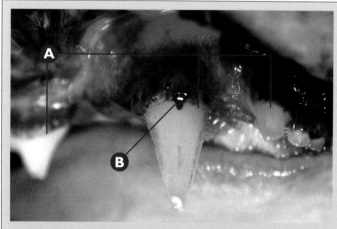

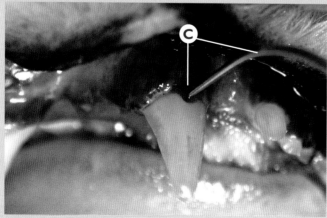

Tooth resorption

Suspicions of stage 2 tooth resorption of RmaxC (104).

Ⓐ From right to left: RmaxI3 (103), RmaxC (104) and RmaxP3 (107).

Ⓑ Suspicions of stage 2 tooth resorption of RmaxC (104).

Ⓒ Image of the suspicions of stage 2 tooth resorption of RmaxC (104) assessed with a dental explorer, with loss of enamel and dentin.

Key diagnostic/treatment points
The use of a dental explorer is truly fundamental to detect small tooth resorption lesions. In this clinical case, a lesion is suspected in the apical third of the crown of RmaxC (104), on the vestibular surface (near the gingival margin); the presence of the lesion can be confirmed using an explorer. Dental X-rays are indicated to assess the true extent of the process, as well as to confirm the stage.

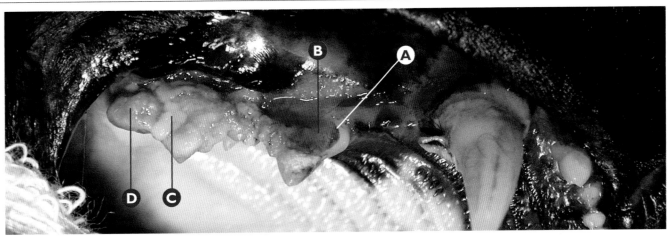

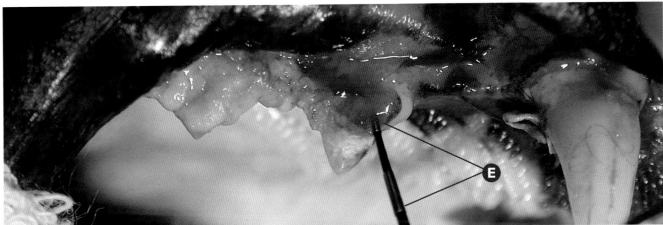

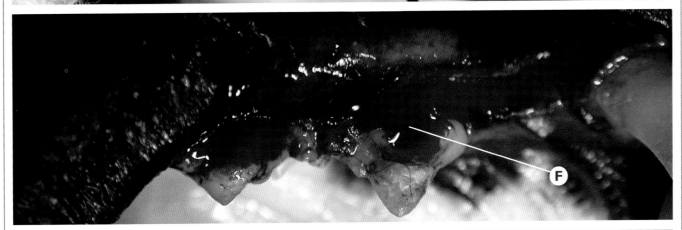

Tooth resorption

Suspicions of stage 3 tooth resorption of RmaxP3 (107).

Ⓐ Suspicions of stage 3 tooth resorption of RmaxP3 (107), with obvious loss of dental tissue (enamel and dentin).

Ⓑ Gingival hyperplasia reactive to the tooth resorption in the vestibular area of RmaxP3 (107).

Ⓒ Plaque index 4 on RmaxP4 (108).

Ⓓ Calculus index 4 on RmaxP4 (108).

Ⓔ Use of a periodontal probe to confirm the depth of the dental destruction under the hyperplastic gingiva.

Ⓕ Confirmation of the suspicions of stage 3 tooth resorption, after checking for pulp exposure and partial removal of the hyperplastic gingiva.

Key diagnostic/treatment points

In tooth resorption, we frequently detect reactive gingival hyperplasia that attempts to cover the dental defect caused by the disease. As a result, on these occasions, it is difficult to determine the stage of tooth resorption macroscopically. Confirmation of the stage by means of dental X-rays is mandatory.

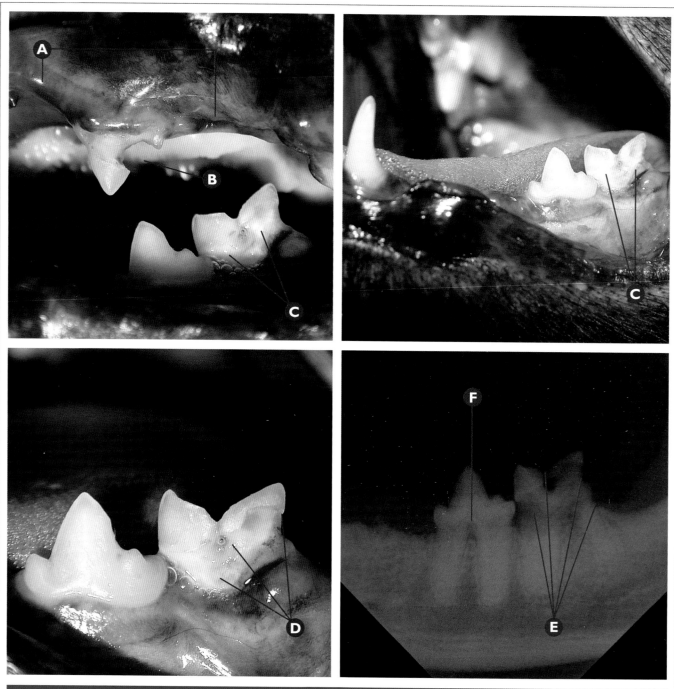

Tooth resorption

Stage 2 tooth resorption of LmandM1 (309).

Ⓐ From right to left: absence of LmaxP4 (208) and LmaxP2 (206).

Ⓑ Suspicions of stage 3 tooth resorption of LmaxP3 (207).

Ⓒ Suspicions of stage 2 tooth resorption of LmandM1 (309).

Ⓓ Close-up of the suspicions of stage 2 tooth resorption of LmandM1 (309).

Ⓔ Dental X-ray: radiological signs compatible with stage 2 tooth resorption of LmandM1 (309).

Ⓕ Dental X-ray: radiological signs compatible with the initial stage of tooth resorption in the furcation area of LmandP4 (308).

Key diagnostic/treatment points

Tooth resorption is frequently underdiagnosed or confused with dental fractures or caries. The literature describes this condition as very common in the oral cavity of domestic felines. The use of a dental explorer is very useful to detect small lesions. In advanced stages, the macroscopic aspect is enough to detect most of the affected teeth. However, dental X-rays are indispensable to determine the true degree of involvement in the entire oral cavity. In many patients, we can detect dental absences, which are often attributable to a stage 5 of this oral disease, due to complete destruction of the dental tissue.

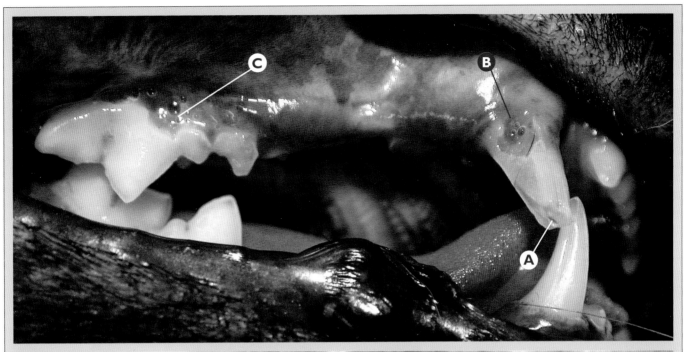

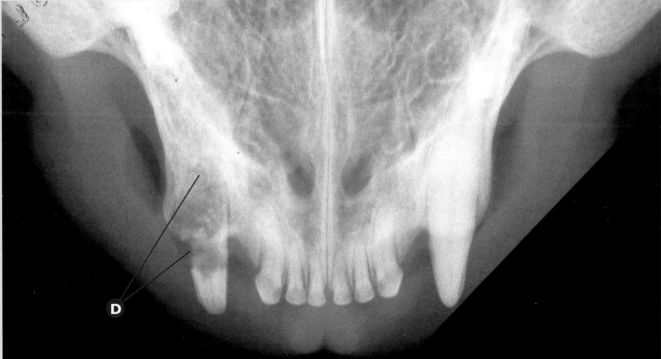

Tooth resorption

Stage 4 tooth resorption of RmaxC (104).

A Complicated crown fracture of RmaxC (104).

B Suspicions of stage 4 tooth resorption of RmaxC (104), due to severe destruction of the vestibular area of the apical third of the crown.

C Suspicions of stage 3 tooth resorption of RmaxP4 (108).

D Dental X-ray: radiological signs compatible with stage 4c tooth resorption due to complete destruction of the root of RmaxC (104).

Key diagnostic/treatment points

Occasionally, especially in the upper and lower canine teeth, the crowns may appear relatively normal macroscopically, while X-rays may reveal that they are completely destroyed by tooth resorption (stage 4). In this clinical case, the complicated crown fracture of RmaxC (104) has probably caused the faster progress of the process.

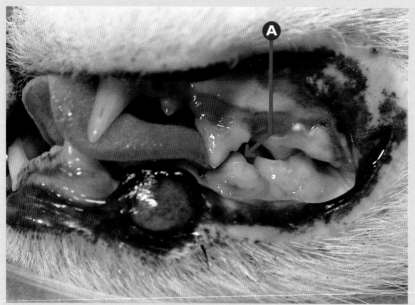

Tooth resorption

Malocclusion in the distal region of the premolars and molars of the left side, suspected to be due to stage 4 tooth resorption of LmaxP4 (208).

Ⓐ Palatal deviation of the mesial area of the crown of LmaxP4 (208), suspected to be due to stage 4 tooth resorption; left vestibular view.

Ⓑ Suspicions of stage 4 tooth resorption of LmaxP4 (208); left vestibular view.

Ⓒ Malocclusion in the distal region of the premolars and molars of the left side, with occlusion of the distal cusp of LmandM1 (309) on the vestibular surface of LmaxP4 (208); left vestibular view.

Ⓓ Image of the palatal deviation of the mesial area of the crown of LmaxP4 (208), due to suspicions of stage 4 tooth resorption.

Ⓔ Calculus index 1 on RmaxP4 (108).

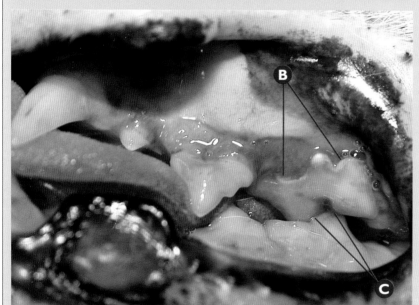

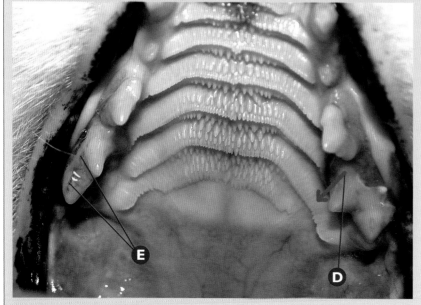

Key diagnostic/treatment points
Occasionally, in cases of tooth resorption and more particularly in advanced stages, deviations and rotations of the dental crowns may occur as a result of root resorption, which causes the tooth to lose its base. As occurs in this case, this leads to malocclusion that prevents the animal from closing its mouth, with the resulting oral pain. To confirm stage 4 tooth resorption, a regional dental X-ray must be taken to detect the advanced degree of dental destruction.

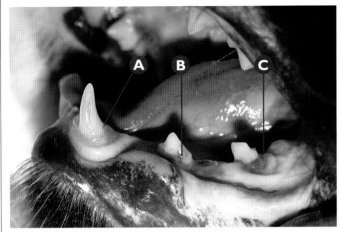

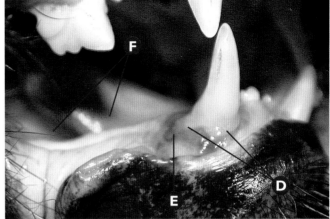

Tooth resorption

Stage 4 tooth resorption of LmandC (304), LmandM1 (309), RmandC (404) and stage 3 lesions in LmandP3 (307).

Ⓐ Suspicions of stage 2 tooth resorption of LmandC (304).

Ⓑ Suspicions of stage 3 tooth resorption of LmandP3 (307).

Ⓒ Suspicions of stage 4 tooth resorption of LmandM1 (309).

Ⓓ Discharge of seropurulent fluid from the gingival margin of RmandC (404).

Ⓔ Gingival index 2 in RmandC (404).

Ⓕ Absence of RmandP3 (407) and RmandP4 (408).

Ⓖ Mandibular abscess/inflammation in the chin area.

Ⓗ From right to left: absence of LmandI1 (301) and LmandI2 (402).

Ⓘ Dental X-ray: radiological signs compatible with stage 4c tooth resorption due to complete destruction of the root of LmandC (304).

Ⓙ Dental X-ray: radiological signs compatible with stage 4c tooth resorption of RmandC (404).

Ⓚ Dental X-ray: radiological signs compatible with stage 4c tooth resorption of RmandI3 (403).

Ⓛ Dental X-ray: radiological signs compatible with stage 3 tooth resorption of LmandP3 (307).

Ⓜ Dental X-ray: radiological signs compatible with stage 4a tooth resorption of LmandM1 (309).

Ⓝ Dental X-ray: radiological signs compatible with mesial root of LmandM1 (309).

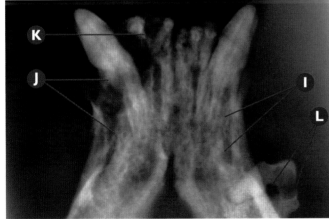

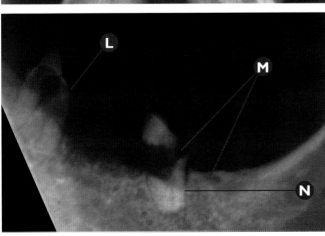

Key diagnostic/treatment points

This clinical case is a clear example of stage 4 tooth resorption of the canine teeth, in which no or only minimal lesions of the crown have been detected during the oral examination; however, there is severe root destruction, detected by means of dental X-rays. Occasionally, we can detect periodontal pockets in the affected teeth with discharge of seropurulent fluid. Treatment will consist of the extraction of the teeth affected by stage 3 and 4 tooth resorption.

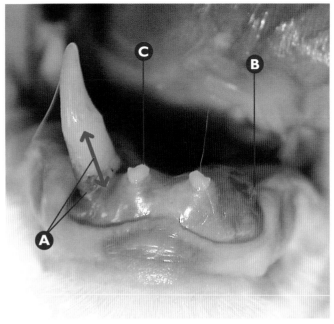

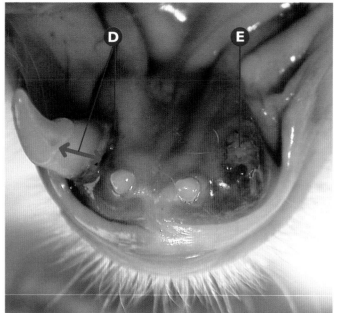

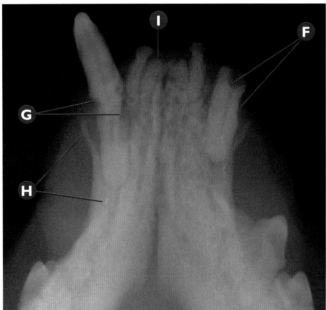

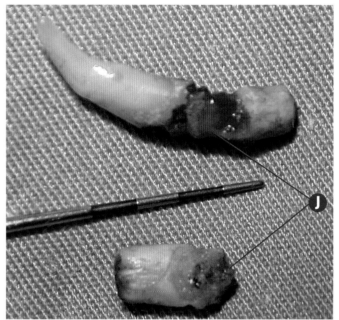

Tooth resorption

Stage 4 tooth resorption of LmandC (304) and stage 2 in RmandC (404).

Ⓐ Stage 4 periodontal disease in RmandC (404).

Ⓑ Suspicions of a retained root of LmandC (304).

Ⓒ RmandI2 (402).

Ⓓ Image of stage 4 periodontal disease in RmandC (404).

Ⓔ Image of a retained root of LmandC (304).

Ⓕ Dental X-ray: radiological signs compatible with stage 4b tooth resorption of LmandC (304).

Ⓖ Dental X-ray: radiological signs compatible with stage 2 tooth resorption of RmandC (404).

Ⓗ Dental X-ray: radiological signs compatible with stage 4 periodontal disease in RmandC (404), due to dental extrusion and expansion of the vestibular bone.

Ⓘ Dental X-ray: radiological signs compatible with a retained root of RmandI1 (401), probably affected by tooth resorption (stage 4b).

Ⓙ Close-up of RmandC (404) and the retained root of LmandC (304), after its extraction.

Key diagnostic/treatment points

Occasionally, we can detect the presence of two very advanced conditions in the same tooth. This is the case of RmandC (404), affected by advanced stages of periodontal disease and tooth resorption. Those teeth affected by stage 3 and 4 tooth resorption must be extracted.

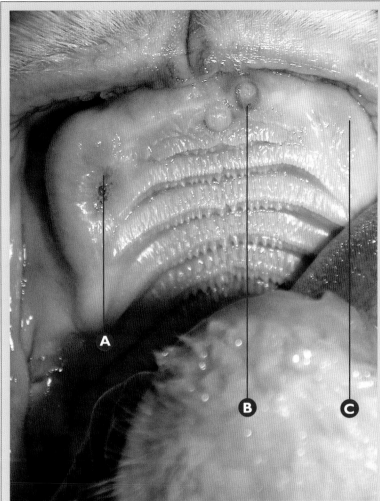

Tooth resorption

Stage 5 tooth resorption of LmaxC (204) and stage 3 in LmaxI1 (201).

Ⓐ Absence of RmaxC (104).

Ⓑ LmaxI1 (201).

Ⓒ Absence of LmaxC (204).

Ⓓ Dental X-ray: radiological signs compatible with stage 5 tooth resorption of LmaxC (204).

Ⓔ Dental X-ray: radiological signs compatible with stage 3 tooth resorption of LmaxI1 (201).

Ⓕ Dental X-ray: radiological signs compatible with absence of RmaxC (104).

Key diagnostic/treatment points

The situation detected in LmaxC (204) is a case of stage 5 tooth resorption. Dental destruction is nearly complete. In the case of LmaxI1 (201), although it seems to be disease-free in the oral examination, the dental radiological study reveals stage 3 tooth resorption, due to the involvement of the cement, dentin and pulp cavity of the tooth.

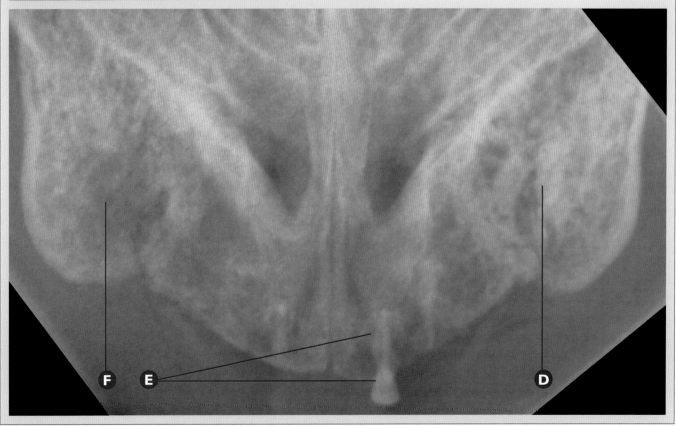

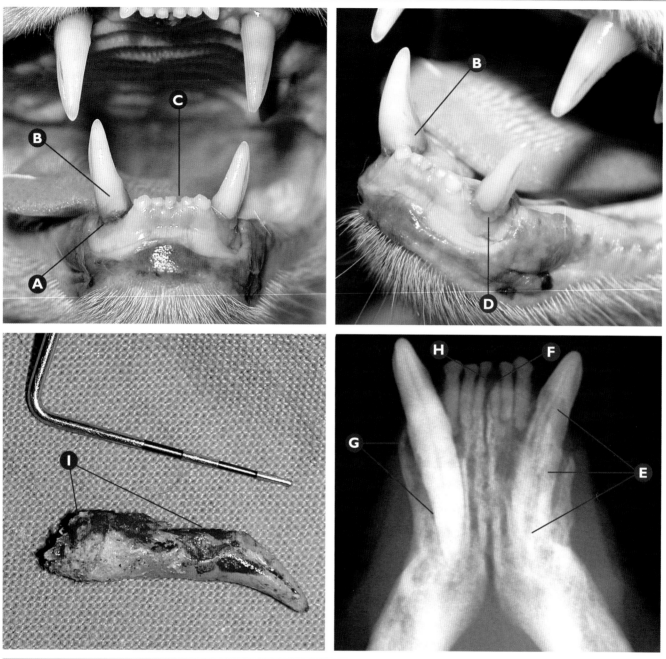

Tooth resorption

Stage 3 tooth resorption of LmandC (304).

A Suspected stage 3 periodontal disease in RmandC (404).

B Dental discolouration in RmandC (404).

C Absence of LmandI1 (301).

D Suspicions of stage 1 tooth resorption of LmandC (304).

E Dental X-ray: radiological signs compatible with stage 3 tooth resorption of LmandC (304).

F Dental X-ray: radiological signs compatible with stage 4b tooth resorption of LmandI1 (301).

G Dental X-ray: radiological signs compatible with stage 4 periodontal disease in RmandC (404), moderate expansion of the vestibular bone, with severe changes to the periodontal ligament in this region.

H Dental X-ray: radiological signs compatible with stage 2 tooth resorption of RmandM1 (401).

I Close-up of LmandC (304), after dental extraction.

Key diagnostic/treatment points

Even in those clinical cases where the lesions detected macroscopically are mild, dental X-rays will provide the necessary information for an accurate determination of the stage of tooth resorption. Those teeth affected by stage 3 tooth resorption (with pulp exposure) must be extracted.

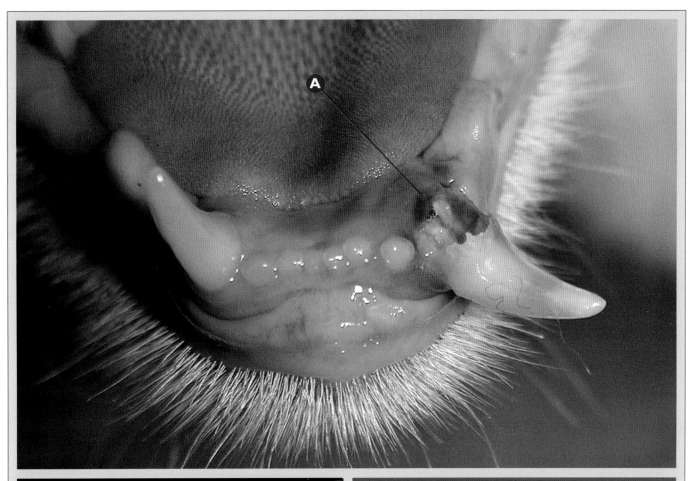

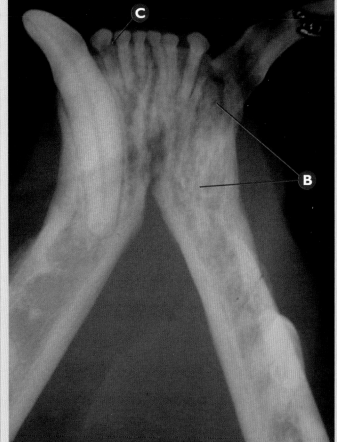

Tooth resorption

Stage 4 tooth resorption of LmandC (304).

Ⓐ Suspicions of a complicated crown-root fracture of LmandC (304).

Ⓑ Dental X-ray: radiological signs compatible with stage 4c tooth resorption due to complete destruction of the root of LmandC (304).

Ⓒ Dental X-ray: radiological signs compatible with stage 3 tooth resorption of RmandI3 (403).

Key diagnostic/treatment points

This clinical case is another typical example of stage 4 tooth resorption of LmandC, with the other canine tooth not affected by this process (RmandC), as seen on the dental X-rays. On those occasions where we detect severe dental fractures with no known previous trauma, tooth resorption must be one of our primary differential diagnoses. Dental X-rays are indispensable to reach a correct diagnosis in these clinical cases. Treatment is based on the elimination of the dental tissue by means of a coronectomy and surgical closure of the gingiva.

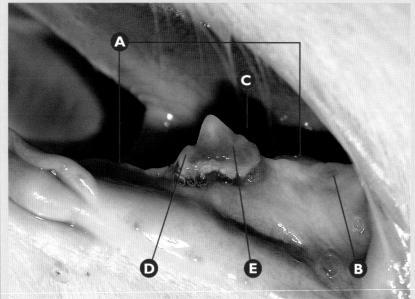

Tooth resorption

Stage 4 tooth resorption of LmandP4 (308) and LmandM1 (309).

A From right to left: absence of LmandM1 (309) and LmandP3 (307).

B Suspicions of a retained root of LmandM1 (309).

C Suspected stage 3 periodontal disease in RmandP4 (308).

D Plaque index 3 on LmandP4 (308).

E Calculus index 4 on LmandP4 (308).

F Close-up of stage 3 periodontal disease in LmandP4 (308).

G Dental X-ray: radiological signs compatible with stage 4c tooth resorption of LmandP4 (308).

H Dental X-ray: radiological signs compatible with stage 4b tooth resorption of LmandM1 (309), with the retained mesial and distal roots.

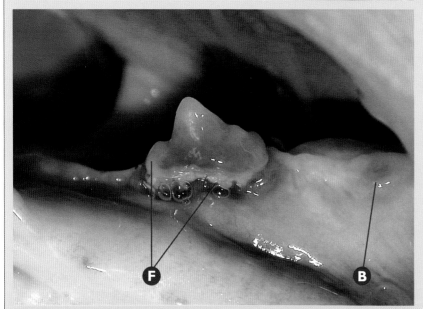

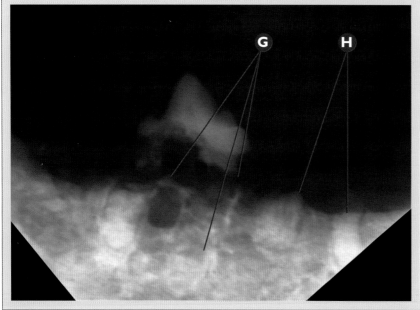

Key diagnostic/treatment points

This is another clear example of the importance of dental X-rays to determine the stage and true condition of the teeth affected by tooth resorption. In spite of our suspicions of advanced periodontal disease in LmandP4 (308), the absence of regional teeth makes us suspect the presence of tooth resorption in this region. Dental X-rays will be essential to assess the true extent of the condition. On this occasion, treatment will be based on the extraction of LmandP4 (308) (crown and mesial root), as well as of the retained roots of LmandM1 (309).

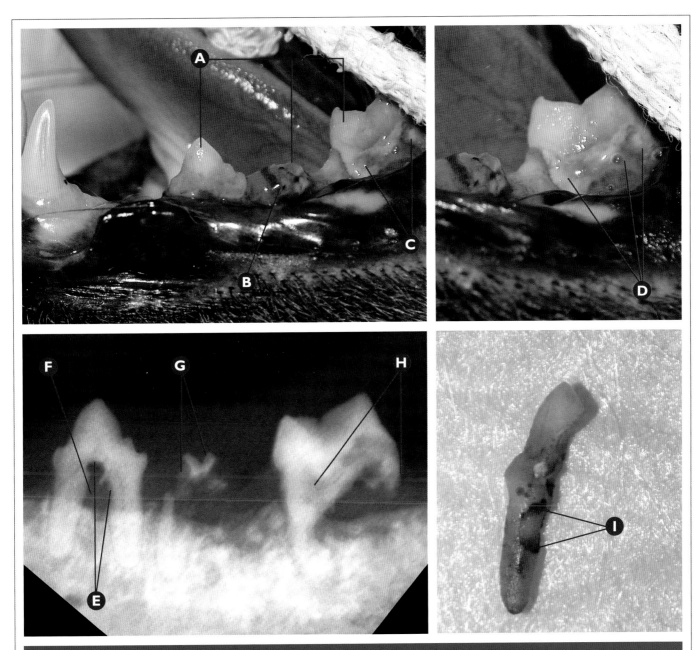

Tooth resorption

Stage 2 tooth resorption of LmandP3 (307) and stage 4 in LmandP4 (308) and LmandM1 (309).

A From right to left: LmandM1 (309), LmandP4 (308) and LmandP3 (307).

B Suspicions of stage 4 tooth resorption of LmandP4 (308).

C Suspected stage 4 periodontal disease in LmandM1 (309).

D Close-up of the suspected stage 4 periodontal disease in LmandM1 (309).

E Dental X-ray: radiological signs compatible with stage 2 tooth resorption of LmandP3 (307).

F Dental X-ray: radiological signs compatible with class 3 furcation in LmandP3 (307).

G Dental X-ray: radiological signs compatible with stage 4a tooth resorption of LmandP4 (308).

H Dental X-ray: radiological signs compatible with stage 4c tooth resorption of LmandM1 (309).

I Close-up of the resorption of the mesial root of LmandP3 (307), after performing the odonto-section of the tooth during its surgical extraction.

Key diagnostic/treatment points
We may observe teeth affected by tooth resorption with a very different macroscopic appearance in the same region, and regional dental X-rays may reveal different stages of tooth resorption. Regardless of the stage of periodontal disease or tooth resorption, treatment of these three teeth is extraction.

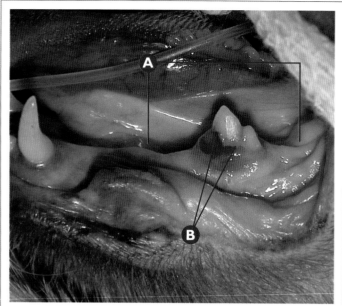

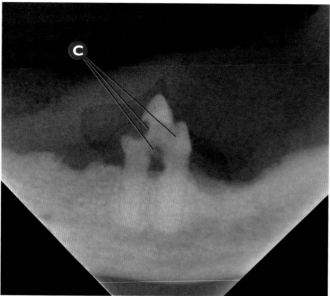

Tooth resorption

Stage 3 tooth resorption of LmandP4 (308).

Ⓐ From right to left: absence of LmandM1 (309) and LmandP3 (307).

Ⓑ Suspicions of stage 3 tooth resorption of LmandP4 (308).

Ⓒ Dental X-ray: radiological signs compatible with stage 3 tooth resorption of LmandP4 (308).

Key diagnostic/treatment points
In this clinical case, the absence of LmandM1 (309) and LmandP3 (307) may be due to their previous extraction, or the final consequence of tooth resorption. In the case of LmandP4 (308), surgical extraction will be the treatment of choice to resolve the process.

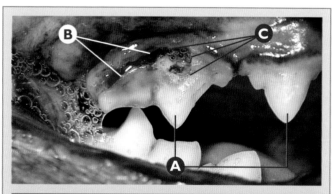

Tooth resorption

Suspicions of stage 3 tooth resorption of RmaxP4 (108).

Ⓐ From right to left: RmaxP3 (107) and RmaxP4 (108).

Ⓑ Suspicions of stage 3 tooth resorption of RmaxP4 (108).

Ⓒ Close-up of the resorption in the vestibular area, in the neck of RmaxP4 (108).

Key diagnostic/treatment points
The use of a dental explorer and dental X-rays will confirm whether this is a stage 3 or 4 of tooth resorption. In both stages the treatment involves the extraction of the teeth, and dental X-rays will inform us of the state of the tooth at the time of the extraction.

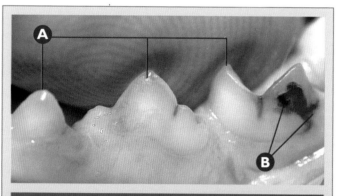

Tooth resorption

Suspicions of stage 3 tooth resorption of LmandM1 (309).

Ⓐ From right to left: RmandM1 (309), RmandP4 (308), RmandP3 (307).

Ⓑ Suspicions of stage 3 tooth resorption of LmandM1 (309).

Key diagnostic/treatment points
In this clinical case, LmandM1 (309) is macroscopically affected by resorption of the neck and crown of the tooth, which is apparently affecting the pulp chamber. The use of a dental explorer and dental X-rays are highly indicated in this clinical case.

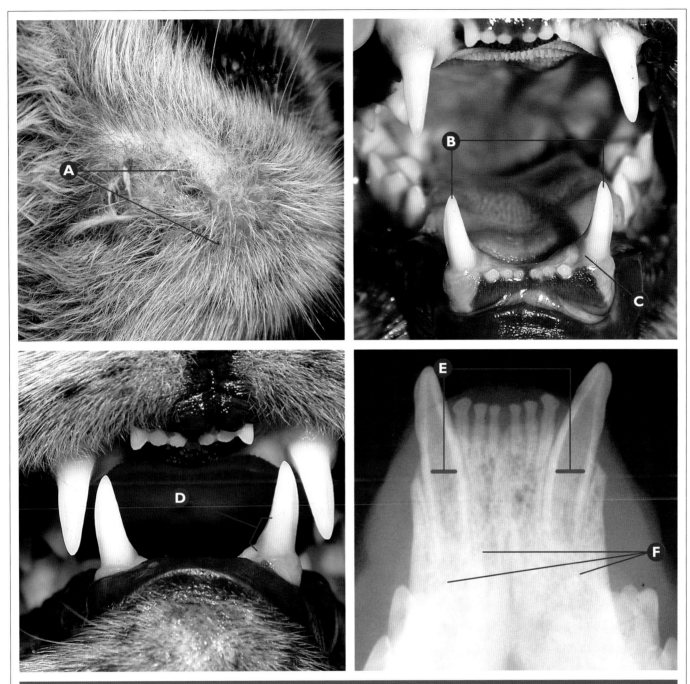

Endodontic disease

Endodontic disease in LmandC (304) and RmandC (404) with pulp necrosis, which has degenerated into a mandibular abscess in the chin area of an adult patient with a history of trauma.

A Severe mandibular abscess in the chin area.

B From right to left: LmandC (304) and RmandC (404), with no macroscopic signs of dental fracture.

C Dental discolouration in LmandC (304).

D Close-up of the dental discolouration in LmandC (304).

E Dental X-ray: (from right to left) radiological signs compatible with endodontic disease due to the wide diameter of the pulp cavities of LmandC (304) and RmandC (404).

F Dental X-ray: radiological signs compatible with areas of moderate diffuse osteolysis.

Key diagnostic/treatment points

Occasionally, in patients that have suffered trauma (especially to the symphyseal area), it is possible to observe an endodontic disease of the canine teeth with no clear signs of periodontal disease or a complicated crown fracture, only dental discolouration in some cases. The trauma has caused an irreversible lesion to the odontoblasts as well as pulp necrosis, which will progress to periapical disease (dental abscess in its last phase).

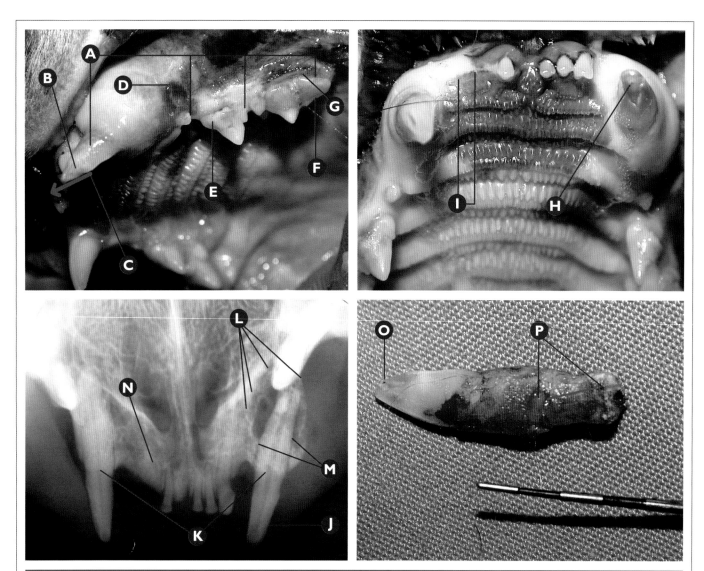

Endodontic disease

Formation of a periapical granuloma at the root of LmaxC (204), which has progressed to an abscess, as a consequence of endodontic disease (complicated crown fracture).

Ⓐ From right to left: LmaxP4 (208), LmaxP3 (207), LmaxP2 (206) and LmaxC (204).

Ⓑ Suspicions of a complicated crown fracture of LmaxC (204).

Ⓒ Mesial deviation of LmaxC (204).

Ⓓ Fistulous tract in the mucosa, apical to LmaxP2 (206).

Ⓔ Plaque index 2 on LmaxP3 (207).

Ⓕ Calculus index 4 on LmaxP4 (208).

Ⓖ Gingival index 2 in LmaxP4 (208).

Ⓗ Complicated crown fracture of LmaxC (204).

Ⓘ From right to left: absence of RmaxI2 (102) and RmaxI3 (103).

Ⓙ Dental X-ray: LmaxC (204).

Ⓚ Dental X-ray: radiological signs compatible with a diameter of the pulp cavity wider than that of RmaxC (104), a radiological sign compatible with endodontic disease in LmaxC (204).

Ⓛ Dental X-ray: radiological signs compatible with a periapical granuloma at the root area of LmaxC (204).

Ⓜ Dental X-ray: radiological signs compatible with osteolysis and an increase of the space of the periodontal ligament of LmaxC (204).

Ⓝ Dental X-ray: radiological signs compatible with stage 5 tooth resorption of RmaxI2 (102).

Ⓞ Close-up of the pulp necrosis in the pulp cavity due to the complicated crown fracture of LmaxC (204), after its extraction.

Ⓟ Close-up of root resorption in LmaxC (204).

Key diagnostic/treatment points

Just like dogs, cats can suffer from endo-perio lesions (type I, II or III). In this case, the most probable aetiology of the process is the complicated crown fracture of LmaxC (204). This causes pulp necrosis and eventually periapical disease, with formation of a periapical granuloma. The periapical granuloma is detected radiologically as an area of diffuse radiolucency with loss of lamina dura. If we do not stop the process, the endodontic disease will cause a periodontic lesion, which in this case is a type I endo-perio lesion. The severe lesion in the periodontal ligament is the most probable cause of the dental displacement due to the loss of dental insertion. Adequate treatment in this clinical case is dental extraction.

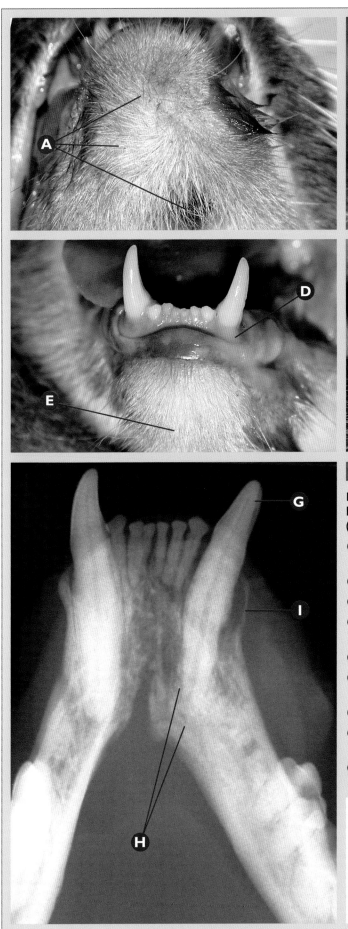

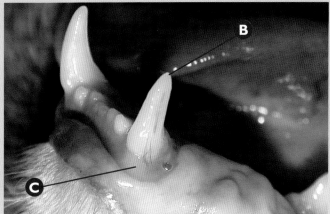

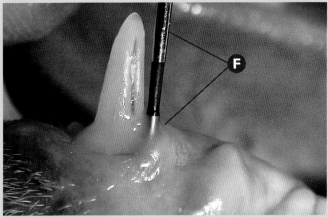

Endodontic disease

Formation of a periapical granuloma at the root of LmandC (304), which has progressed to an abscess, as a consequence of endodontic disease (type II endo-perio lesion).

A Severe mandibular abscess distal to the symphyseal area, with a fistula draining to the exterior.

B LmandC (304).

C Purulent exudate draining from the subgingival area of LmandC (304).

D Purulent exudate draining from the subgingival area of LmandC (304); rostral view.

E Image of the severe mandibular abscess.

F Periodontal pocket greater than 10 mm in the distovestibular area of LmandC (304), determined using a periodontal probe.

G Dental X-ray: LmandC (304).

H Dental X-ray: radiological signs compatible with periapical disease in LmandC (304), with areas of osteolysis and root destruction.

I Dental X-ray: radiological signs compatible with expansion of the vestibular bone in LmandC (304).

Key diagnostic/treatment points

In endo-perio lesions, type II in this clinical case, there is periapical disease due to the changes to or lesion of the periodontal ligament, which eventually causes changes to the bone tissue and periapical tissue and probably also subsequent endodontic disease (pulp necrosis). The presence of a periapical granuloma may develop, such as in this clinical case, into a dental abscess. We must perform a differential diagnosis with tooth resorption. Adequate treatment includes extraction of the affected tooth.

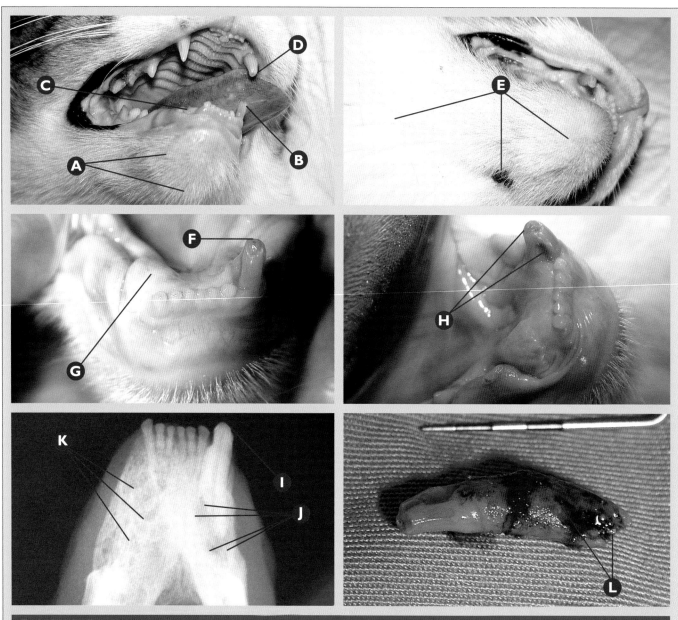

Endodontic disease

Periapical granuloma at the root of LmandC (304), which has progressed to an abscess, as a consequence of a complicated crown fracture of the tooth that has caused endodontic disease (type II endo-perio lesion).

A Severe mandibular abscess in the symphyseal area.

B Suspicions of a complicated crown fracture of LmandC (304).

C Suspicions of absence of RmandC (404).

D Complicated crown fracture of LmaxC (204).

E Close-up of the severe mandibular abscess with drainage to the exterior through a fistula on the left side.

F Complicated crown fracture of LmandC (304), with exposure of the pulp (black colour typical of pulp necrosis).

G Absence of RmandC (404).

H Close-up of the dental discolouration and complicated crown fracture of LmandC (304).

I Dental X-ray: radiological signs compatible with a complicated crown fracture of LmandC (304).

J Dental X-ray: radiological signs compatible with a periapical granuloma and destruction of the dental tissues in the root of LmandC (304).

K Dental X-ray: radiological signs compatible with absence of RmandC (404), with bone reaction.

L Close-up of the root of LmandC (304), after its extraction.

Key diagnostic/treatment points

In endo-perio lesions, type I in this clinical case, there is periapical disease due to the complicated fracture of the tooth, which causes pulp necrosis that progresses in an apical direction. A periapical granuloma eventually forms and progresses into a dental abscess. Dental extraction is the adequate treatment.

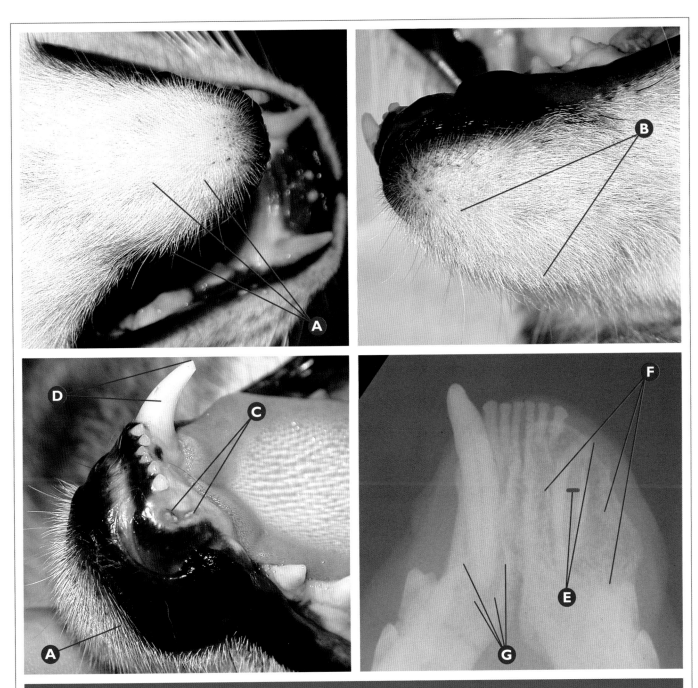

Endodontic disease

Formation of a dental abscess around the root of LmandC (304), as a consequence of a complicated crown-root fracture of the tooth that has caused endodontic disease (type I endo-perio lesion). Periapical granuloma at RmandC (404).

A Severe mandibular abscess in the chin area, mainly on the left side.

B Close-up of the severe mandibular abscess in the chin area.

C Complicated crown-root fracture of LmandC (304).

D Suspicions of enamel fracture of on RmandC (404).

E Dental X-ray: radiological signs compatible with a complicated crown-root fracture of LmandC (304), old fracture with a wide pulp chamber.

F Dental X-ray: radiological signs compatible with severe osteolysis in the region near the retained root of LmandC (304).

G Dental X-ray: radiological signs compatible with a periapical granuloma at RmandC (404).

Key diagnostic/treatment points

In type I endo-perio lesions due to a complicated fracture of the tooth (old fracture), there is endodontic disease (pulp necrosis) that eventually progresses into a periapical granuloma and dental abscess. In RmandC (404), we detect radiological signs compatible with periapical disease, of an unknown origin, although it could easily be related to the process developed on the left side. Adequate treatment of LmandC (304) is dental extraction.

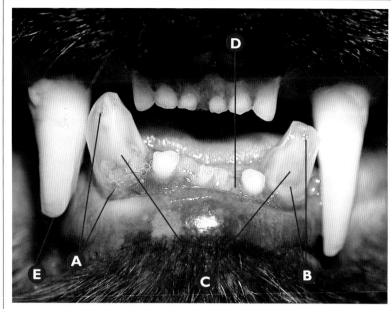

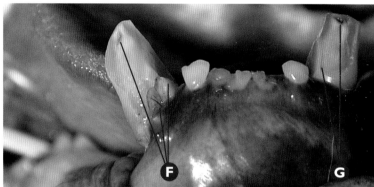

Endodontic disease

Formation of a periapical granuloma at LmandC (304) and RmandC (404) as a consequence of a complicated fracture of both teeth (type I endo-perio lesion).

A Complicated crown-root fracture of RmandC (404).

B Suspicions of a complicated crown fracture of LmandC (304).

C Discolouration of LmandC (304) and RmandC (404); the most probable cause is endodontic disease.

D Absence of LmandI2 (302).

E Suspicions of a complicated crown fracture of RmaxC (104).

F Close-up of a complicated crown-root fracture of RmandC (404).

G Confirmation of a complicated crown fracture of LmandC (304).

H Dental X-ray: radiological signs compatible with a periapical granuloma at RmandC (404).

I Dental X-ray: radiological signs compatible with a severe lesion of the periodontal ligament and stage 2 tooth resorption of RmandC (404).

J Dental X-ray: radiological signs compatible with a periapical granuloma at LmandC (304).

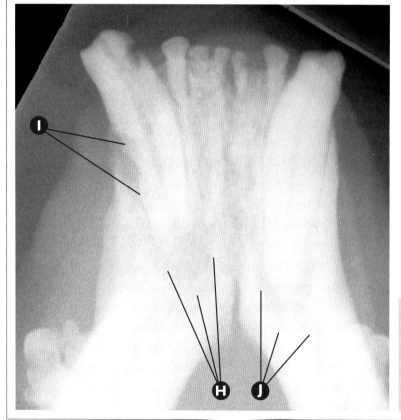

Key diagnostic/treatment points
Both complicated crown fractures and complicated crown-root fractures degenerate into pulp necrosis without appropriate treatment. This could be the cause of the dental discolouration. If in spite of the pulp necrosis, no treatment is performed, a periapical granuloma will eventually form in the tissues that surround the apex of the tooth.

References

AMERICAN VETERINARY DENTAL COLLEGE. Veterinary Dental Nomenclature. Journal of Veterinary Dentistry, 2007, 24(1); pp. 54-57.

AVDC BOARD. Veterinary Dental Nomenclature. Recommendations from the AVDC Nomenclature Committee adopted by the American Veterinary Dental College Board. 2007.www.avdc.org.

BELLOWS, J.E., DUMAIS, Y., GIOSO, M.A., REITER, A.M., VERSTRAETE, F.J. Clarification of Veterinary Dental Nomenclature. Journal of Veterinary Dentistry, 2005, 22(4); pp. 272-279.

BOJRAB, M.J., THOLEN, M. *Small Animal Oral Medicine and Surgery*. Philadelphia: Lea & Febiger, 1990.

CAMBRA, J.J. *Manual de Cirugía periodontal, periapical y de colocación de implantes*. Mosby Harcourt Brace Publishers International, 1996.

CATTABRIGA, M., PEDRAZZOLI, V., WILSON, TG. JR. The conservative approach in the treatment of furcation lesions. Periodontology 2000, 2000, 22(1); pp. 133-153.

COHEN, S., HARGREAVES, K. *Pathways of the Pulp*. 9th edition. Elsevier Mosby, 2006.

COLLADOS J. Técnica de Extracción en Sobrecrecimiento de Incisivos en Lagomorfos. Pequeños Animales, Revista Informativa Veterinaria. 2004, Nº 49; pp. 47-55.

COLLADOS, J. Odontología Veterinaria III. Exodoncia, Traumatología Oral y Endodoncia. ARGOS, Revista Informativa Veterinaria. Jul-Ago 2001.

COYNE, K.P., DAWSON, S., RADFORD, A.D., CRIPPS, P.J., PORTER, C.J., McCRACKEN, C.M., GASKELL, R.M. Long-term analysis of feline calicivirus prevalence and viral shedding patterns in naturally infected colonies of domestic cats. Veterinary Microbiology, 2006, Nov 26: 118(1-2); pp.12-25.

DEFORGE, D.H., COLMERY III, B.H. *An Atlas of Veterinary Dental Radiology*. Iowa State University Press, 2000.

EUBANKS, D.L. Oral Soft Tissue Anatomy in the Dog and Cat. Journal of Veterinary Dentistry, 2007, 24(2); pp. 126-129.

FLOYD, M.R. The Modified Triadan System: Nomenclature for Veterinary Dentistry. Journal of Veterinary Dentistry, 1991, 8(4); pp. 18-19.

FONSECA, R.J., BAKER, S.B., WOLFORD, L.M. *Cleft/Craniofacial/Cosmetic Surgery*. 1st edition. Philadelphia: W.B. Saunders Company, 2000.

GARDNER, D.G. An orderly approach to the study of odontogenic tumours in animals. Journal of Comparative Pathology, 1992, 107(4); pp. 427-438.

GARDNER, D.G. Dentigerous cysts in animals. Oral Surgery, Oral Medicine, Oral Pathology, Oral Radiology, and Endodontology, 1993, 75(3); pp. 348-352.

GARDNER, D.G., DUBIELZIG, R.R., McGEE, E.V. The so-called calcifying epithelial odontogenic tumour in dogs and cats (amyloid-producing odontogenic tumour). Journal of Comparative Pathology, 1994, 111(3); pp. 221-230.

GATINEAU, M., EL-WARRAK, A.O., MANFRA MARRETTA, S., KAMIYA, D., MOREAU, M. Locked Jaw syndrome in Dogs and Cats: 37 Cases (1998-2005). Journal of Veterinary Dentistry, 2008, 25(1); pp. 16-21.

GAUTHIER, O., BOUDIGUES, S., PILET, P., AGUADO, E., HEYMANN, D., DACULSI, G. Scanning Electron Microscopic Description of Cellular Activity and Mineral Changes in Feline Odontoclastic Resorptive Lesions. Journal of Veterinary Dentistry, 2001, 18 (4); pp. 171-176.

GOAZ, P.W., WHITE, S.C. Oral Radiology Principles and Interpretation. 3rd edition. St. Louis: Mosby, 1994.

GORREL, C. Odontología Veterinaria en la Práctica Clínica. Servet, 2006.

GORREL, C., LARSSON, A. Feline odontoclastic resorptive lesions: unveiling the early lesion. Journal of Small Animal Practice, 2002, 43; pp. 482-488.

HARVEY, C.E. Shape and Size of Teeth of Dogs and Cats-Relevance to Studies of Plaque and Calculus Accumulation. Journal of Veterinary Dentistry, 2002, 19(4); pp. 186 -195.

HARVEY, C.E., EMILY, P.E. Small Animal Dentistry. Mosby-Year Book Inc., 1993.

HENNET, P.R. Chronic Gingivo-stomatitis in Cats: Long-term Follow-up of 30 Cases treated by Dental Extraccions. Journal of Veterinary Dentistry, 1997, 14(1); pp. 15-21.

HILLSON, S. Teeth. 2nd edition, 2005.

KERTESZ, P.A. Colour Atlas of Veterinary Dentistry and Oral Surgery. London: Wolfe, 1993.

LLENA-PUY, M.C., FORNER-NAVARRO, L. Anomalía morfológica coronal inusual de un incisivo. Diente evaginado anterior. Medicina Oral, Patología Oral y Cirugía Bucal, 2005, 10; pp. 13-16.

LOBPRISE, H.B., WIGGS, R.B. Anatomy, Diagnosis and Management of Disorders of the Tongue. Journal of Veterinary Dentistry, 1993, 10(1), pp. 16-23.

LOMMER, M.J., VERSTRAETE, F.J.M. Concurrent oral shedding of feline calicivirus and feline herpesvirus 1 in cats with chronic gingivostomatitis. Oral Microbiology and Immunology, 2003, Apr 18(2); pp. 131-134.

LYON, K.F. Dental home care. Journal of Veterinary Dentistry, 1991, 8(2); pp. 26-30.

NEWMAN, M.G., TAKEI, H.H., CARRANZA, F.A. Carranza's Clinical Periodontology. 9th edition. W.B. Saunders Company, 2002.

OKUDA, A., HARVEY, C.E. Etiopathogenesis of Feline Dental Resorptive Lesions. Veterinary Clinics of North America: Small Animal Practice, 1992, 22; pp. 1385-1404.

PETERS, E., LAU, M. Histopathologic examination to confirm diagnosis of periapical lesions: a review. Journal of the Canadian Dental Association, 2003, 69(9); pp. 598-600.

PETTERSSON, A., MANNERFEL,T. Prevalence of Dental Resorptive Lesions in Swedish Cats. Journal of Veterinary Dentistry, 2003, 20 (3); pp. 140-142.

POPOVSKY, J.V., CAMISA, C. New and emerging therapies for diseases of the oral cavity. Dermatologic Clinics, 2000, 18(1); pp. 113-125.

POULET, H., BRUNET, S., SOULIER, M., LEORY, V., GOUTEBROZE, S., CHAPPUIS, S. Comparison between acute oral/respiratory and chronic stomatitis/gingivitis isolates of feline calicivirus: pathogenicity, antigenic profile and cross-neutralisation studies. Archives of Virology, 2000, 145(2); pp. 243-261.

REGEZI, J.A., SCIUBBA, J.J., JORDAN, R.C.K. *Oral Pathology: Clinical Pathologic Correlations.* 4th edition. St. Louis: Saunders, 2003.

REITER, A.M., MENDOZA, K.A. Feline odontoclastic resorptive lesions: An unsolved enigma in veterinary dentistry. Veterinary Clinics of North America: Small Animal Practice, 2002, 32; pp. 791-837.

REUBEL, G.H., HOFFMANN, D.E., PEDERSEN, N.C. Acute and chronic faucitis of domestic cats; a feline calicivirus-induced disease. Veterinary Clinics of North America: Small Animal Practice, 1992, Nov 22(6); pp. 1347-1360.

ROUX, P., BERGER, M., STOFFEL, M., STICH, H., DOHERR, M.G., BOSSHARD, D., SCHAWALDER, P. Observations of the Periodontal Ligament and Cementum in Cats with Dental Resorptive Lesions. Journal of Veterinary Dentistry, 2005, 22(2); pp. 74-85.

SALYER, K.E, BARDACH, J. *Atlas of Craniofacial Surgery.* Philadelphia: Lippincott-Raven Publishers, 1999.

SAN ROMÁN, F. *Atlas de Odontología en Pequeños Animales.* GRASS Editions, 1998.

SLATTER, D. *Tratado de Cirugía en Pequeños Animales.* 3ª Edición. Intermedica, 2007.

THONGUDOMPORN, U., FREER, T.J. Prevalence of dental anomalies in orthodontic patients. Australian Dental Journal, 1998, 43(6); pp. 395-398.

TUTT, C., DEEPROSE, J. AND CROSSLEY, D. *BSAVA Manual of Canine and Feline Dentistry.* 3rd edition. London: Blackwell Publishing, 2007.

VERSTRAETE, F.J.M. *Self-Assessment Colour Review Of Veterinary Dentistry.* London: Manson Publishing, 1999.

VERSTRAETE, F.J.M., TERPAK, C.H. Anatomical Variations in the Dentition of the Domestic Cat. Journal of Veterinary Dentistry, 1997,14(4); pp. 137-140.

WIGGS, R.B., LOBPRISE, H.B. *Veterinary Dentistry: Principles and Practice.* Lippincott - Raven, 1997.

WOLF, H.F., RATEITSCHAK-PLUSS, E.M., RATEITSCHAK, K.H. *Color atlas of dental medicine. Periodontology.* 3rd edition. Georg Thieme Verlag, 2005.

Alphabetic index

Published by Servet editorial - Grupo Asís Biomedia S.L.